D0857080

The Real Race

The Real Race

BY SKIP WILKINS AND JOSEPH DUNN

JCP

CORP. OF VIRGINIA

Virginia Beach, Va.

Library of Congress Catalog Number 80-85152

ISBN No. 0-938694-04-9

Copyright ©1981 by Skip Wilkins and Joseph Dunn. All rights reserved.
No parts of this book may be reproduced in any form without written
permission from the publisher and, where applicable, the authors.

JCP Corp. of Virginia
214 40th Street
P.O. Box 814
Virginia Beach, Virginia 23451

Book and dustjacket design by W. Bradley Miller
Dustjacket photography by Ronn Maratea
Authors' photos on back cover and inside flap by Mike Combs

Biblical quotations are from *Holy Bible: New International Version*, copyright ©1978 by The New York International Bible Society. Used by permission of Zondervan Bible Publishers and from *The New English Bible*,
Copyright © The Delegates of the Oxford University Press and the Syndics
of the Cambridge University Press 1961, 1970. Reprinted by permission.

Acknowledgements

It became an impossible task to mention all of the families, friends
and people who have helped me in my life and with this book.

I am grateful to all of them and I hope that they are proud of what they
have helped one person do with his life.

Skip Wilkins
March 11, 1981

Ice Cream and Courage

We met in an ice cream parlor. It was as unlikely a place for me to be as was the reason that took me there. I was a newspaperman then and given more to a quick and convenient sandwich than dessert at a distant place. I had been asked to meet Skip Wilkins; he was seeking advice on writing a book that he felt it was time to write.

I was much taken with him when we met. He was attractive and articulate. Unassuming, yet assured. And he was terribly excited about life. He easily made me forget that he was in a wheelchair.

My guidance to him about the book didn't take long; I'd never written one. I gave him the names of some people I thought could help him and took my leave.

Courage. That's what I thought on my way back to the office. I've met a young man with a lot of courage.

We came together again a year later — in the spring of 1979. I had just put 22 years of newspapering behind me and he had his book ahead of him. I helped a little with an outline of the book and we talked a lot about what he wanted to say. Then I left for a place with sunshine before starting out in a new direction.

When I returned to Virginia Beach, I was asked to help Skip write this book. It was an invitation to a longer journey than the two of us could have imagined.

I've met a lot of people along the way. Some personally. Some indirectly. They've contributed generously — checking records and memories — to these pages. The most loyal and the most helpful person has been a very bright young woman named Bonnie Mattiko. She kept us, especially me, going when other duties became frustrating distractions and turned into long delays. If she enjoys the fruits of her loyalty, her help, her suggestions and her plain hard work, that's a big reward.

Over the months, I've met with Skip's wife Daphne and his family and they have relived for me some terrible and some touching experiences. They, too, have become special people.

I've gotten to know Skip Wilkins perhaps as well as anyone outside his family. I think that I'm counted among his friends. He is listed among mine. That's been the big benefit.

And there's something else that's come out of all this: an understanding that you never know what you'll find or where you might find it. After all, courage isn't an everyday flavor in an ice cream parlor.

Joseph Dunn
March 9, 1981

To my family,
To my wife,
And all to the glory of God

S.W.

Contents

The Real Race

Part One

With each rhythmic forward thrust of his arms, Skip Wilkins propelled his wheelchair toward the indoor sports stadium and pumped more adrenalin through his body.

He felt good. It was not a typically English day. The sun had been warm at 7:30 when he fidgeted through the announcements at the team's morning meeting. Now he could feel its heat on his shoulders as he took his place in the procession for the opening ceremonies.

He looked around. The athletes from 29 countries were an impressive sight. The colors of their uniforms and their nations' flags were brilliant in the midday sun. His team, the United States team, looked as smart and as crisp as any, he thought.

The stadium entrance was packed with families and friends of the athletes and spectators from the neighboring towns and villages. He tried to locate Daphne in the crowd. He spotted her and she waved. As the procession of athletes began to move inside, he looked ahead, where the coaches were grouped, and picked out Wayne Whitley. He smiled, thinking how nervous and excited Daphne and Wayne had been earlier that morning. His wife and his coach. Always with him. He wondered if they really understood how important they were to him.

The procession entered the stadium, moved past the reviewing stand and came to a stop in a large formation for the opening ceremonies.

Sir Ludwig Guttmann began to speak. He recounted the history of Stoke Mandeville and the international games. He told how the Stoke Mandeville Hospital had been established by the British as a rehabilitation center for the maimed of World War II. He told the story of the birth of the competitive athletic program to give the war's crippled a novel incentive as they tried to regain their spirit, their dignity and their sense of worth. The program had been successful and it had been broadened in the years since 1948 to unite thousands of paralyzed men and women in sportsmanship and competition.

Skip was aware that the story he was hearing was really the story of the man who was speaking. Poppa, never Sir Ludwig, was what the athletes called him. He was a German doctor who had gained a reputation as one of his country's finest brain surgeons. He had come to England in 1939 as a Jewish refugee. In 1944 he had opened the Spinal Injuries Center at Stoke Mandeville Hospital. It had been Poppa who had envisioned sports as a key to rehabilitation of the war wounded.

It had been Poppa who had guided the program at Stoke. When he started in 1948, the program consisted of a few wheelchair games on the front lawn. Now it included the large indoor stadium and an Olympic-style village that was Skip's world for the present.

Skip felt a catch in his throat and swallowed hard at the words that now came from the speaker's platform:

"I declare the 1979 International Stoke Mandeville Games for The Physically Disabled to be open," Sir Ludwig's voice boomed.

The loudspeakers sent forth strains of the British national anthem which were quickly drowned out by a unified cheer from the massed athletes.

1

Weber. The big, strong German. Always there. Always the real competition. Always a little bit better each year. Just out of reach.

Well, not this year. No. This was Skip's year. Skip's mind flicked from item to item down his personal checklist for the shot put.

Then it was time. He spotted the German, already warming up, and he began to calculate each move he would make.

Skip Wilkins had begun his ritual of competition.

He rolled past Weber at the throwing area and slowed for a moment. They nodded. Each offered a half-smile, polite but cool. They knew that they were it — the only serious contenders for the gold. Once more, the battle was between them. It was an unspoken message, a jockeying for advantage. Part of the ritual.

Skip worked his way out of his warmup jacket and began hefting a practice shot. He checked the lineup. He would throw after the German. Another break. Like the weather. Unusually warm for England, even in July. He rolled to a spot under the scoreboard. He had made a note of the location when he and Daphne had scouted the throwing area days before. He would be able to face Weber when the German was in the throwing circle. In past meets, he'd been to the side, studying his opponent's form and the technique. Today he wanted to be seen. Eye to eye on each throw.

Weber's name was called over the loudspeaker. After his chair was locked in place with the restraining chains, the German looked out at the throwing area. Skip was in Weber's line of sight and their eyes met. Then Weber turned to his work. The official handed a shot to him. He raised it several times, getting the feel of the lead ball. He nodded to the official. Then he settled into his throwing position, pulling the shot close to his neck. He continued to work the shot slowly around in his hand, seeking the most comfortable position. Then he was still. Skip could see his chest heave as he took the deep breath before the throw.

Weber's first try easily put him in first place in the trials. Skip had expected that. No question that the contest was between the two of them. One would take the gold, the other would place second and take the silver. The rest of the athletes would battle for the third spot.

Weber threw again. Slight improvement.

Then he made his final throw in the trials. Skip didn't look for the adjust to the weight. He returned it and took the second shot. It, too, felt slightly heavier than two kilos, but it was lighter than the first. That happened. No two shots were identical. He nodded to the official who retreated with the first shot.

Skip inched his torso toward the front of the chair. He reached his left hand behind the left chair handle and hooked his thumb beneath the handle. It was a natural position now, but it had come only after months of work and experimentation with Wayne. It gave Skip maximum leverage. He positioned the shot more comfortably in his hand and tucked it under his chin.

At that moment Skip Wilkins, from his head down to his upper chest, looked like any shot-putter. He had broad, muscular shoulders and a strong neck. His throwing position was classic.

"Come on, Skip. This is it," he told himself. The muscles in his left arm tightened all the way down to the thumb that was hooked beneath the chair handle. In one fluid motion, he pulled his body toward the throwing area with his left arm and thrust his right arm up and out and released the shot. It was a good, clean throw, but Skip didn't think that it traveled far enough to dislodge Weber from first place. The crowd's reaction told him otherwise when the shot thudded into the ground. The second throw felt good and he knew the third had to be close to Weber's distance.

Skip rolled out of the circle.

"What's your best mark?" the official asked. Before Skip could recall the figure, his marks were called over the loudspeaker.

"Wilkins. U.S.A. First throw, 4.92 meters. Second throw, 5.09. Third throw, 5.12."

It wasn't a personal record, but it was more than enough for the trials.

Skip wheeled to Wayne and Daphne. He didn't try to hide his excitement. He was in first place. First place in world competition. He was two-tenths of a meter in front of Weber. He did some quick conversion math. About nine inches. That was a solid difference if Weber had given his throws everything that he could. Skip suddenly realized that he was standing in first place for a world gold medal. Weber would have only three more tries, in the finals, to overtake him. The roles were reversed for the first time. Weber had to catch him now. Had Weber held back? If so, how much had the German saved for the finals?

Skip rolled to a shaded area. He watched the remaining five competitors. None came even close to Weber's throw.

He headed for the dorm and rest. He was still caught up in the results of the trials. He lay down, but sleep wouldn't come quickly. He tried to force his mind to slow down, but it wouldn't. It kept toying with the prospect of winning the world title. For a while, he gave up trying to suppress the thought. It was too pleasant. But he knew that it was a dangerous thought. "Don't start wearing medals before you win them," he told himself.

He began to unwind. Sleep was coming, but it would have to wait long enough for him to think back over the past few days of July 1979, the days that had brought him to within reach of his biggest athletic goal . . .

Daphne Elizabeth Wilkins.

Skip liked the sound of her name. He never tired of gazing at her, especially when she was unaware of his attention, as she was now. She was chatting with one of the score of well-wishers in the terminal at Norfolk International Airport. He always broke into a smile when he looked at her. Even when he was upset with her, which was seldom. She had come into his life when things were rough, rougher than he could have imagined they would be for a young man of 23. He and Daphne had married nearly three years after they met, and they were making it together now when many of their friends were spending time and money and emotion in the offices of counselors and divorce lawyers.

Skip thought to himself how attractive Daphne was, even beautiful. Her mouth, barely touched with makeup, was parted in a smile. Her eyes, hazel, were sparkling. Her head was tilted back, just slightly, so that her loosely curled hair just touched her shoulders. She had fussed about her hair before the trip.

He watched her as she moved. She was tall and slender, the figure of a model; graceful. As always, she was neatly dressed.

Striking, Skip thought to himself. That was the word that he had chosen long ago to describe his wife. Striking, and so important to him. He was thankful that she would be with him on the trip.

"Ladies and gentlemen," came the voice over the microphone. "Allegheny's Flight One Eighty-Nine for Baltimore is now ready for boarding. Please extinguish all smoking materials and have your boarding passes ready for the agent. Will those passengers with small children, passengers in wheelchairs and anyone else needing assistance please come to the aisle on my left. We will board you first."

Patsy Wilkins bent to kiss her son on the cheek. It was a warm, affectionate kiss, not the kind that most 29-year-old sons would comfortably accept in a public place. But the Wilkins family had made it through the roughest of times by being close; they were a loving family, never hesitant to show affection.

"You and Daphne be careful. Take care. We'll be praying for you," she said. Then she added, as always, "And have a good time."

Tommy Wilkins had been watching his son with undisguised pride.

"Do good, son," he said. "You know we're with you. And call us if you can." His hand came down firmly and gently on Skip's shoulder.

Stepping back, he glanced at Wayne Whitley. "Watch out for the chair, Wayne," Tommy said.

Then came Shirley. Skip's sister wrapped her arms around his neck and kissed him on each cheek. She was 20, but she had the irrepressible excitement of a child.

"You all have a good time. Aren't you excited? We'll be praying for you." Her three thoughts poured out in a single stream of enthusiasm.

Other well-wishers extended hands to Skip as he headed toward the aisle. When he reached the plane's door, he stopped. Wayne and a flight attendant reached down to lift him out of his wheelchair. Wayne wrapped both of his arms around Skip's chest and locked his hands. He explained to the young man in the blue-and-red Allegheny uniform how to lift Skip's legs free of the foot plates. Once Skip had cleared the chair, the two men carried him onto the plane. Another flight attendant folded the chair and took it down to the runway level for storage in the baggage compartment. After Skip was settled, Wayne would check on the chair. It had become part of his boarding routine.

Daphne had preceded Skip to the seat with his cushion and two bulging flight bags. Wayne checked on the chair. It was stowed aboard.

The plane taxied down the runway and Skip and Daphne Wilkins and Wayne and Diane Whitley were on their way to Baltimore, then New York, then London. Their final destination was Wendover, England, home of the Stoke Mandeville games, the site of the 1979 world competition for disabled athletes.

Only in the terminal at Baltimore did Skip become bored and edgy. They had more than an hour layover. He occupied the idle time watching the endless scurrying of people through the airport. He often wondered what the other people-watchers thought of him. He believed that he was nice looking. He took pride in his appearance. He was careful about his clothes, selecting traditional cuts that could be altered easily to fit him neatly and comfortably.

He had a narrow muscular face, deep-set and penetrating brown eyes and a well-shaped, full mouth. His hair was light brown, thick but soft, and he parted it casually just off the center. He had a strong athletic neck. Not the bull neck of a college or professional football player. It had some length and grace. If anything, his shoulders were larger than perfect proportions would have required. The rest of his body, clothed, was well proportioned to his head and shoulders. But he, and those who had seen him in competition, knew that the body was slender and without the muscle and the flesh that people, seeing him from the neck up, would expect. He glanced down at his chest. His eye caught the patch on his jacket. It was a coat of arms, in the shape of a shield. A wheelchair, embroidered in red on a white field, was in the top right of the shield. Seven vertical red-and-white stripes, similar to the stripes of the U.S. flag, were in the lower left. Across the middle of the shield was a broad stripe of blue. Embroidered across that blue field were the three white letters: USA. It was the emblem of the United States wheelchair sports team.

Two years before his invitation to become a member of the U.S. team, back in 1974 when he first started to compete, he found himself assigned to a group of athletes with a different kind of designation, the designation of 1A. That was his medical classification for sports. Class 1A. He belonged to that group now. He always would. It included the most severely damaged of the athletes. The classification included individuals who had suffered damage to the fourth, fifth or sixth cervical vertebrae. The injury, by definition, had to result in complete or incomplete quadriplegia affecting the use of both hands, weakening the triceps and causing severe weakness in the trunk and lower extremities which, in turn, interfered significantly with trunk balance and the ability to walk. The classes that followed, the 1Bs and 1Cs, had increasingly greater use of arm muscles and fingers, and more strength in the trunk and lower extremities.

The voice over the public address system interrupted Skip's thoughts and announced the flight to New York. The journey to England resumed.

The seven days at Wendover had been a kaleidoscope of minor problems, long practices and mounting pressure.

The bed was too high. That was the first problem. Skip spotted that as soon as he entered the dorm. He long ago had learned to judge distance with precision. An inch could make for a mountain. It had taken an hour of practice, under Wayne's watching, to feel confident that he could transfer from chair to bed without help.

He and Weber played a cat-and-mouse game for the first two days. The grapevine had confirmed that both had come to the games. It also speculated endlessly about who would win. The two had finally greeted each other after the opening ceremonies on Sunday. Each of them, with gestures and a few basic words of English, protested that the other was the athlete to beat. Skip left that brief encounter with Weber without the tinge of intimidation that he had always felt in the past when he first saw the huge German.

Skip was alternately deflated and exhilarated when the games actually began. He had lost his singles table tennis match to a German newcomer. He had won the bronze in the club throw. Weber had won the silver and McCoole, the Irishman, had taken the gold. The medal helped. It was Skip's first of the games and it gave him a boost to know that he had contributed to the U.S. effort. The elation was short-lived. He made the finals in the discus, but failed to win a medal. He was eliminated, as he expected to be, in the first heat of the 60-meter race. He simply didn't have the strength for racing. He opted to sit out the lawn bowling, always a competition when the games were in England. He and Rod Vleiger had battled the world's No. 1-ranked table tennis players to the wire before losing in team table tennis, a combination of singles and doubles matches. The U.S. pair had won the bronze, but Skip knew that he had played the best table tennis of his career. It was enough, just before the last day — the day of the shot put — to restore much of his confidence.

"Good games so far," Skip thought as he closed his eyes to sleep before the finals. "If I can just hold on in the shot . . ."

Wayne's voice brought Skip out of his sleep. It was 4:40 p.m. Time for his last test of the 1979 season.

A large crowd had gathered for the finals. Athletes from every country were lined behind the circle. There were only four finalists in the event. Skip's three competitors already were working with their coaches to stretch and warm their muscles. He and Weber again exchanged nods. No half smiles this time. Skip found a spot out of sight from the throwing circle. It was Weber now who would have to apply the pressure. Skip wasn't going to make it easy for him.

The fourth-place man was in the circle and beginning to position himself for his first throw. The thought of being No. 1 in the world suddenly was broken by a strange and illogical possibility: suppose the fourth-place or the third-place man had been holding back? Suppose one of them beat Weber and Skip? Skip watched the shot as it left the thrower's hand and began its arc. Before it landed Skip knew that the fourth-place man might move up one position, but he would not come close to Skip or Weber. The second throw, then the third, followed the arc of the first and landed within inches of his first effort. He hadn't improved his standing.

Now the third man began his positioning for his first throw. Again Skip thought of the improbable. Suppose? But there wasn't any supposing. The No. 3 man improved his own mark slightly, but remained well behind Weber.

Skip tried to remain calm, but couldn't. Daphne rested her arm across his shoulder. He reached up and rested his hand on hers. His face, as he looked up at her, reflected sheer excitement. His eyes were wide and his mouth was all smile.

Weber was in the circle, taking a lot of time to get his chair positioned.

"Hurry up," Skip said in a slight voice. He was anxious. He wanted to know immediately how much better he would have to throw to beat the German. Weber's first throw was a poor one. "Maybe he didn't hold back," Skip started to tell himself. But Skip knew better. Weber had been too anxious on the first throw and had released too soon. The throw was well behind his distance in the trials.

It seemed that hours passed as Weber readied for his second throw. Skip squirmed in his chair. The whole area was silent. There wasn't a spectator who even whispered to another as Weber launched his second throw. It was not a long one. Again Weber had let the shot go an instant too soon. Skip knew from his own experience that the pressure was a big factor. Weber had to know, before that second throw, that he had only two chances to keep his title. Now he had only one chance left.

Skip's mouth went dry. He wanted to call out, yell, do anything to break the tension. He wasn't sure that he could watch the last throw. It could mean as much to him as it could mean to Weber. Skip wanted to turn away, to avoid the possible sight of the shot soaring beyond his ability to match it or to beat it. But his competitive instincts overpowered his nerves. He watched as Weber leaned forward, brought his weight to the back of the chair and snapped his body forward and extended his arm. The throw looked good. The crowd sighed in admiration as the shot reached the highest point of its flight.

"That's the big one," Skip said in the direction of Wayne as he began to raise and lower his right arm, holding a shot.

When Wayne didn't respond, Skip looked at his coach. Suddenly Wayne was jumping up and down and grinning.

"You've done it. You've beaten him. He's 4.91. You've won it," Wayne said with the first show of excitement that Skip had seen on the trip.

Skip turned toward the head official. The figures were being called out for Weber's last throw. "Weber. West Germany. Four. Point. Nine. One. Meters."

It was over. Skip had become the world champion in the shot put. He had been better than Weber. He was the best in the world. Skip felt tears in his eyes. He swallowed and smiled. More tears came. Daphne was leaning down, hugging him. She was crying, too. She couldn't say anything. Neither could Skip. They looked at each other, then at Wayne. It was their moment. It had been a long time in coming.

Skip lay in bed, wide awake. He was just beginning to settle down from the emotion-packed day. His mind went back to the field and the shot put. He had, after bringing himself under control, moved into the circle after Weber and completed his three throws. The throws weren't required, but there was always the chance that he might break the world-record distance of 5.82 meters. He hadn't done that. He had improved over his best throw in the trials and he ended up with a final winning distance of 5.16 meters.

That evening Skip and Daphne had joined the others with the U.S. team for dinner in the Red Lion Inn. It had been a relaxed and friendly gathering. The athletes had been able to unwind as they celebrated the team's achievements and marked the end of the games.

After dinner, Skip had called home to tell his family what he had done in the games. He had relived all of the excitement on the field as he recounted to his father the victory in the shot.

Now, before drowsiness finally began to overcome him, Skip's thoughts turned to God. He was thankful for the victory. He thought back over the last few years. He thought about faith and how faith alone sometimes carried him, his family, and Daphne through the difficulties of recuperation and rebuilding.

Skip Wilkins had a feeling of great satisfaction now, but he knew that he owed his success and his happiness to those around him and to God.

2

Tommy Wilkins slowly returned the telephone receiver to its place. His thoughts were on the conversation that he had just concluded with his son and his hand, by instinct, found its way to the telephone set on the table by the sofa.

He leaned back and relaxed his muscular frame into the sofa and closed his eyes.

A gold medal. A gold medal in world competition. The best. The very best in the entire world. His son. His son who would spend the rest of his life in a wheelchair. His son whom the family had nursed and prayed away from death. His son had won a world gold medal.

Tommy Wilkins, still strong and handsome at 50, still touched by the outdoors life of his long-ago athletic years, relished the solitude. His wife would be home soon from her hostess job at the hospital and he would tell her the news. She would be glad for him and happy for everyone and, most of all, she would remain calm because she had always believed that God willed all events, even the accident, for His own larger purpose. Right now, Tommy savored the time alone. He wanted to indulge himself in the pride that swelled inside him for his son and for the family and what the six of them had done together to bring Skip to this point in his life.

He began thinking back through his life. Skip's homecoming from the rehabilitation center in Fishersville, Virginia. The carpentry work to modify the house to accommodate a wheelchair and a paralyzed son. The accident. The exciting high school years when Skip had starred in football and track. The raising of a son and three daughters. Skip's birth that had marked a new beginning for Tommy as a mature husband and a responsible father. The problems he and Patsy had overcome in their young marriage.

His mind kept flipping back, finally stopping in the years of his youth in Norfolk.

Tommy had been born to a comfortable life. His father had worked for Seaboard Railroad and had acquired numerous residential real estate properties. As a small child, he lived in a large brick house with a brick wall around it. He remembered big birthday parties with friends and their mothers in the yard and the pony that his dad had bought for him. He must have had everything that a child could want in his early years.

But the aura of wealth faded quickly. When Tommy was 4, his father died. His mother tried hard to keep things together, but she was a poor manager of wealth. Soon the land and the several homes that they owned were sold so his mother could continue to live without working.

During the next seven years Tommy stayed for long periods of time with different relatives, although he always returned to his mother. There was no male influence in his life and, for that reason perhaps, he spent much of his schooltime in the principal's office for his antics in class. His grades remained good and his conduct was more mischievous than delinquent. As his frame and his strength grew, so did his daring. He was always the first to accept a challenge, to dive from the railroad trestle above the river, to ride a bicycle off a homemade ramp.

He was introduced to athletics in the way that most 10-year-old boys of his generation were introduced. His friends played their games on a nearby field that was uneven underfoot, but smooth enough to rough-house. One day an older boy appeared with a football and Tommy Wilkins quickly became a standout as a sandlot running back. He enjoyed being pursued. When his team didn't have the ball, he enjoyed the prospect of physical contact. He liked to tackle and didn't mind being tackled.

His mother married again, to a soldier, and the family was transferred to Washington, D.C., as the prospect of war neared.

Tommy was into everything then except the classroom. He took to the boxing ring with success in Golden Gloves competition. He became an accomplished swimmer and a proficient tumbler. He was increasingly absent from school. He skipped classes when it suited his personal schedule. His mother became a frequent visitor to the principal's office and Tommy just as frequently promised to do better. But he didn't or he couldn't or he wouldn't.

Finally he persuaded his mother to allow him to quit high school and enroll in a vocational school. His initial venture into radio electronics was unsuccessful and he found his way into a business course. Before he could prove that he was equal to the task, his mother packed them up and moved back to Norfolk. Tommy's stepfather had been ordered overseas and his mother wanted to return to familiar places and people.

He returned to school and his natural athletic ability carried him to the list of stars in football and track. He remained a mild discipline problem in the classroom, but was a long way from serious trouble. His mother now was in the process of separation from her soldier husband. It had little effect on Tommy. His life was too full of athletics, friends and daredevil stunts.

Tommy's athletic endeavors soon introduced a new element into his life: girls. He was 16 and a mainstay of a community league football team that practiced at city park. One afternoon he noticed two girls on the sidelines watching the team scrimmage. The one who caught his eye was Patricia Wilbern. She went to Granby, the school he had first attended in Norfolk.

It wasn't long before he was sitting on her front stoop in the afternoons and they began to do things together on the weekends. He found the courtship enjoyable. There were hot dog roasts, hayrides and movies.

They saw a lot of each other, but he was still his own person. He picked up jobs to earn spending money and he continued to strengthen his independence. He didn't consult Patsy when he and two friends decided to quit school and go to Florida. The idea was like so many that appealed to Tommy. Spur of the moment. Expression of independence. He worked for two weeks in a drugstore in Florida before he even called Patsy to tell her where he was. She asked him to come back. He said no, but the next day, as suddenly as he had decided to leave home, he caught a bus and returned to Norfolk and to a steady relationship with Patsy Wilbern.

The homecoming was short lived. He was soon bored with the idea of school and he was restless. So three days after his 17th birthday, Tommy Wilkins joined the U.S. Army. He went into the paratroopers because of its reputation for being tough, daring and the best. He took his basic training at Ft. Benning, Georgia, and later was assigned to Ft. Bragg, North Carolina.

At first he enjoyed the challenge and the exhilaration of jumping out of planes. He also began to sense some direction in his life. He returned to the school books under Army auspices and passed the General Education Development Tests, receiving the equivalent of a high school diploma. His relationship with Patsy that had continued through letters was maturing and becoming serious. They talked, in a general way, of marriage sometime in the future. Patsy was the reason that Tommy took his leaves to go back to Norfolk.

Two years with the paratroopers were enough, however. He had relished the life and the reputation that came with it for a while, but it, too, became a routine. At 19, he returned to Norfolk and re-entered school under the GI Bill.

His mother had remarried while he was in the Army and Tommy moved into the apartment with her and his second stepfather, but they had little to do with each other. Tommy, as always, went his own way. Soon he was racing motorcycles and cars, first in neighboring North Carolina and Maryland, then Pennsylvania. He was making money and a reputation of sorts at racing, and he was making mild trouble for himself from time to time with speeding violations on city streets.

He and Patsy saw each other often. They talked about marriage, but it was always something that was going to take place sometime in the future. Tommy was not sure that he wanted to be pinned down by anything or anyone.

An automobile accident changed his mind. They were together one night, riding with two other couples when the car left the road and overturned. Patsy was taken to the hospital with cuts and a back injury. The accident triggered a sense of responsibility in Tommy. He wanted to take care of Patsy. A short time later he asked her parents for permission to marry her. They were reluctant. Patsy was 16 and had not finished high school. But they, too, had married young and they could find no reason to deny their daughter what she wanted.

They were married on October 2, 1948. Patsy was two months past her 16th birthday and Tommy was 19. He gave up racing and quit school to run a gas station seven nights a week. Patsy got a job with the telephone company and gave up any idea of finishing high school. They rented an apartment. But it became evident quickly that they didn't have enough money to be independent so they moved into Patsy's parents' home.

Tommy's job bothered him because it was routine. He started feeling cramped in his in-laws' house. His friends came to see him frequently at the gas station and their freedom made him yearn for his own. He would stay out drinking with them in the early morning hours after he finished work, arriving home to sleep just as Patsy left for her job. In a brief four months after their marriage, the strain and the discord were obvious to almost anyone who knew the young couple. To complicate matters, Patsy was pregnant. She developed kidney problems and was sick frequently. The pregnancy and illness added more worry to Tommy, who already was reeling under his sudden excursion into responsibility for someone other than himself.

He was upstairs one morning, sitting in their room, when his mother-in-law knocked and came in.

"Tommy, I've got to talk to you. I've waited, but you haven't settled down. You know that Patsy is sick and worried. You know she's your wife. But you don't seem to care. Your carrying on is killing her," Mrs. Wilbern said.

She was emotional as she lectured her young son-in-law.

"You're killing her. That's what you're doing. It just can't go on like this. I wish . . . I just wish you'd leave if you can't change your ways."

Tommy knew that she was right. Within 30 minutes he had packed clothes, left the house and moved in with an aunt. He didn't think about calling Patsy. He knew that her mother would have told her by now, and it was best for everyone if he just got out of their lives, he thought.

He quit work at the gas station and took a series of jobs whenever he needed money. He picked up his life the way he had lived it before he and Patsy had married. He was out with his friends at night after work, when he worked. He still was not happy. Restlessness became aimlessness. He went through the motions of living. The jobs, the partying. He performed the same empty ritual over and over, hoping old habits would serve each new day. But they didn't. He missed Patsy. He couldn't be sure that returning to her would answer anything, but he knew that what he was doing held no answer for him.

He visited Patsy occasionally and kept up with her through relatives and mutual friends. As the time came close for the baby to be born, they were drawn together again.

The birth of his son brought him happiness. The child was named after him — Alfred Thomas Wilkins Jr. — although Patsy had nicknamed their baby Skippy. The infant was healthy and so was his wife. Something in Tommy's life had gone well. He even overcame the awkwardness he had felt in being around his mother-in-law. Mrs. Wilbern was kind and pleasant toward him and they began talking.

The after-dinner conversations usually turned to religion. Mrs. Wilbern always had been a devout woman, but it was something new with Patsy. She had become deeply religious during their separation. She went regularly to church and prayed for her life and the life of their son. Tommy didn't understand much about the reason for the change in his wife, but he knew that she was more serene and more confident about her life and her future.

The influence in the Wilbern home had an effect on him. One Sunday with Patsy, he ventured into church for the first time since he had been sent to Sunday School as a child. He began to ask questions, self-consciously at first, then with a desire to learn.

He realized that he did not have a purpose in his life. He had tried and failed to latch on to anything lasting: athletics, motorcycles, cars, paratroopers, school.

He began to learn from Mrs. Wilbern about Bible passages that held out the promise of comfort and peace as a Christian. She was patient in explaining the meaning of the words and how they had helped her. He slowly realized that he wanted to try this life, that he wanted, as Mrs. Wilbern had done, to make a decision for Christ.

That decision was made one evening in the Wilbern home; it came quietly and without drama. Mrs. Wilbern and Tommy were discussing passages from the Book of Romans. They had just finished the passage:

> *"That if you confess with your mouth 'Jesus is Lord' and believe in your heart that God raised Him from the dead, you will be saved."*

Tommy turned to his mother-in-law.
"What do you really have to do, Mrs. Wilbern, to be saved?"
She sensed his seriousness.
"Why don't you let me call Eddie to come over? He's doing Christian lay work and he probably can explain it better than I."

Eddie Hutcheson, Mr. Wilbern's half-brother, soon arrived. He explained to Tommy that there was no magic in such a decision.

"If you would like to make a decision for Christ here, quietly, you can do that, Tommy." Eddie opened the Bible and turned to the passage in Romans that Tommy and Mrs. Wilbern had been discussing.

The two men were alone in the living room.

"Just ask the Lord to come into your heart, Tommy."

Tommy asked. He was quiet for a few moments, then he said a silent prayer.

"Lord, please come into my heart. I want to be a better person."

That was the beginning for Tommy Wilkins.

He prayed. He prayed hardest to lead a better life and to provide a better life for his family. He applied for jobs and he was hired at the Norfolk Naval Air Station as an apprentice electrician to work on aircraft. He moved his family into a small apartment.

Patsy found someone to take care of Skip during the day and she returned to work at the phone company.

It was difficult at first; there was still little money. But Tommy had put his drinking and his aimlessness behind him and he was determined to become a good provider for his wife and his son.

3

The door to the Wilkins' home opened, then quickly and quietly shut. Tommy's thoughts instantly flashed back to the phone call from Skip.

"Skip called. We heard from Skip," he said.

He looked at his wife as she sat down across from him. She was still a pretty woman. Short sandy hair in a loose permanent. A touch of gray was beginning to show. It added to her attractiveness. Her hazel eyes widened at the news. She was beautiful to him when he had met her and she was beautiful to him now across the room.

"What did he say? Are they all . . . " Patsy asked.

Tommy's words rushed out before she could finish the question.

"They're fine. Just fine. He won the gold. He beat the German in the shot. How 'bout that? He won the gold."

Her smile widened. She knew how proud her husband felt.

"Oh, Tommy, can't you see? Can't you see how at one time things looked so grim? You can truly thank God for everything that's happened," Patsy said.

"Patsy, you know there's no way I can ever be thankful for the accident. I wish it hadn't happened. But you're right. I am thankful for the way it's all turned out. I am thankful for that."

They sat together in silence for a moment, each thinking his own thoughts about their son's victory. Then Tommy began to relay all of the details of the competition that Skip and Daphne had told him over the phone.

After a while he pulled himself up from the sofa and headed for his workshop in the garage. He occasionally spent time refurbishing the items that he hunted down in junk shops and at auctions. He liked to work with his hands and the garage had become his place whenever he wanted some time alone.

Patsy sat quietly in the den. She had given a prayer of thanks, and was thinking of her son. Skip's years of hardship and his victory in England gave her reason to pause, too. She knew that she could not appreciate the physical training and the athletic ability that had brought the gold medal to Skip. She did, however, understand how important this event was to her and to the whole family. It had been a long time since she had thought about her life.

Her growing-up years were happy ones. Her parents indulged her at

every opportunity. At 13, she could count among her girlhood posses-
sions a diamond ring, a typewriter and every piece of clothing that she
wanted. Her parents had married when they were both young — her
father was 19 and her mother, 14. They met on a blind date. It was an
unusual match. Patsy's mother came from a strict and religious family.
They had little money. Her dad's family had been well off and he was a
partygoer.

He worked for a brewery and he was a diligent and responsible
employee during the week. But by the time Patsy was a teenager, he had
taken to drinking on the weekends. He was never abusive at home, but
he did tend on those occasions to be remote from his wife and daughter.
Patsy's mother, as time passed, took more and more comfort in her faith
and her Bible.

It was that same faith that got Patsy through her early years of
marriage when she and Tommy were so young and stubborn. They both
had been terribly spoiled as children. She couldn't understand his restlessness and lack of responsibility. A call from his friends for a round of
beer drinking or a night of cards brought his quick and enthusiastic
response in those early days. She was home alone many nights.

Patsy had felt fear when the doctor, looking joyful and happy for
her, told her that she was pregnant. She knew that she and Tommy were
not ready for a child. They couldn't handle their own responsibilities.
Tommy reacted more maturely than she thought he would. He was glad,
he had said, and he hoped that the child would be a boy. But he wanted
more than anything to have a healthy baby. Soon there were doubts
about the health of the child and the mother. Patsy developed serious
and recurring problems with her kidneys. She often was unable to get
out of bed. She had to give up her job before she had planned. Money
became a bigger and bigger problem.

It was then that she began to have long talks with her mother about
her unhappiness. At first her mother initiated the talks, but soon she was
pouring out her troubles and her fears and her concerns about her marriage. She loved Tommy Wilkins, but the two of them were not good for
each other. Her mother was deeply involved in trying to hold her own
life together at the time. She was constantly reading the Bible and
attending church services. She didn't try to force her views on Patsy and

she never mentioned them to her own husband. Yet Patsy saw her mother change over the months. Serenity replaced agitation. Tenderness replaced superficial concern. She was at peace with her life. She explained to Patsy that she had found the Lord, that she had put her life in His hands.

Tommy had left and Patsy's loneliness and worry stirred her to seek what her mother had found. She read the Bible, asked questions of her friends at church and spent time in long conversations with John Dunlap, her minister at Tabernacle Church. Patsy, pressured by a longing for her husband and by a need for comfort, gave her life to the Lord. She promised, too, that her child would be the Lord's.

The birth of their son brought about the first change in Tommy, she thought. He seemed less cocky or sure of himself. He cared about his son. He seemed to be settling down. She was delighted when Tommy asked if he could accompany her to church.

She remembered vividly the night that Tommy gave his life to the Lord. He had done it in his own way and in his own time, not in the church, but in the Wilbern home.

Things weren't perfect between them after that night, but they were together as a family again. It was a beginning. Tommy got a job and he gave up drinking and smoking. He managed to withstand perhaps the toughest personal assault of all — ridicule from his old friends for his sudden change in attitude.

Both of them still had strong wills and streaks of stubbornness. But the arguments became narrowly focused and never strayed into personal hurt.

The family had grown stronger and larger. After Skip came three daughters, Linda in 1951, Karen in 1956 and Shirley in 1958. The life of each child had been dedicated to the Lord. Tommy had continued to work at the Air Station, taking civil service examinations and moving up through the ratings, from a full aircraft electrician, through a variety of posts involving aircraft repair and maintenance, to an Equipment Specialist, managing programs on the use of government equipment.

God had been good to them, she thought. Even with Skip's accident. She knew that Tommy would never agree with her, but she believed that there had been a purpose in the tragedy.

She thought of Skip, now on his way with Daphne to visit Holland before coming home. She remembered the prayer she had offered when he was born, promising that she would give this child of hers and Tommy's to the Lord.

Every day of her life since Skip's birth, she had reminded herself that her son's life belonged to God.

4

The parking lot outside Norfolk General Hospital's emergency room was full. Tommy Wilkins pulled his car to a halt in a "No Parking" zone. He was barely conscious of his hurried look to see that he wasn't blocking anyone as he reached back to shut the car door.

For the second time in his life, he was in Norfolk General. The first time had been a visit that was attended by apprehension and joy. It was the trip on a pleasant evening in September 1949 to see his newborn son for the first time.

There was only fear in this visit on a balmy afternoon, June 12, 1967. His mouth was dry, his heart was pounding and his mind was ticking through endless possibilities of what he might find inside. Again he was coming to this hospital to see his son. But this time there had been an accident. Patsy's call, short, concise and controlled, indicated that Skip might be seriously hurt.

Tommy Wilkins looked down at his son lying on the examining table. A soiled, wet sheet, once white and neatly pressed and folded in its appointed place in the ambulance, covered his son's body up to his neck.

Tommy Wilkins clenched his teeth and called up all of his strength and self-control. He reached down and clasped his hand over his son's and looked into the young man's terrified eyes.

"Skip . . . Son . . . You've got . . . You've got a broken neck."

Tommy battled against the emotion that was trying to take control. He raged inside at what he had been told, at the words he had just spoken to his son. But he wouldn't crumble. He wouldn't yield. He would battle from this moment to see his son well and whole again. He would never quit. Above all, he would never let his son know how much sickness and how much pain had come with the sentence he had just spoken. He wanted desperately to throw himself on his son's helpless body, but he maintained his composure and squeezed hard on his son's hand.

"I have to go now. For a while. But your Uncle Bill will be with you. And your mom and I will be with you in a little while."

Tommy retreated slowly from his son's side. He took a deep breath

and walked softly out of the small and orderly examining cubicle where
his son lay with a broken neck. He let the tears come.

"Why?
"Why?
"Why, God?
"How?
"How?"

Tommy's mind swept back to Patsy's phone call. He tried to remember everything that had happened in the past hour. He hoped that an
answer to the "Why?" and the "How?" might be wrapped up in the
chain of events that had left him drained and so very afraid.

The phone call had come at his office about 1:30 p.m., shortly after
lunch. He could remember every word because the conversation had
been brief.

"Tommy . . . Tommy, I think you better leave work if you can.
Skippy's been hurt. Honey, I think he's hurt real bad. It's a neck injury,
they say. Please hurry. He's at Virginia Beach General. In the emergency room."

"I'll leave right now," Tommy said. He couldn't absorb what he
had just heard.

Tommy turned to Bill Johnson, at the desk behind him.

"Bill, I've gotta leave. Skip's been hurt. Maybe real bad." He took
his jacket from the coat rack and was gone.

Halfway on the 20-mile drive to the Beach, an ambulance passed
him heading toward Norfolk. He wondered who was inside. Was it
Skip? Would they move him? Would Patsy have found the time to call?

He drove on, knowing only the words of Patsy's message. Emergency room. Virginia Beach. Tommy arrived and told the emergency room
nurse who he was.

"I'm sorry, Mr. Wilkins. Your son was transferred to Norfolk
General," she said. "They left about an hour ago. Your wife tried to
call you. But you had left. Can I do anything for you? I imagine that
they're already at the hospital."

"Did my wife ride with him, do you know?"

"Yes. Yes, she did."

Tommy returned to the car and to the highway that he had just traveled. Fear and the queasiness in his stomach were rising as he turned into the Norfolk General lot. He thought he was going to be sick when he saw the sign. "Emergency Room Entrance."

After Tommy left the examining cubicle and his son's side, Skip was moved from the emergency room into the operating room.

The bright lights were gone. Skip was aware of the change. The lights had made his eyes tired.

The voices and the noises were clearer for longer periods of time. The lights were yellow now.

He heard his Uncle Bill's voice.

"Skip." Bill Butler waited for acknowledgement. Skip's eyes turned to look at him.

"Skip. This is Dr. Neal. He's going to help you. Can you listen to him for a minute?" William E. Butler, 65, a general surgeon and Tommy Wilkins' uncle, slowly moved out of Skip's view. In his place was another man. He was a young, short man with glasses. He stuttered ever so slightly.

The man bent to Skip.

"Skip. I'm Dr. Neal. We're going to have to do a few things to you to straighten your neck. They won't hurt. But I want to tell you what we're going to do."

Skip murmured, indicating that he heard and that he was listening.

"We're going to put some things in your head to hold your neck straight. We'll have to shave your head. You'll feel a prick perhaps. And you'll hear the sound of a drill. It won't hurt. I want you to just relax as much as you can."

Skip murmured again.

Richard K. Neal Jr., a young Norfolk neurosurgeon who was rapidly gaining an excellent reputation, was now behind Skip's head. There was movement, but Skip couldn't see. Then he felt a slight tugging sensation at his scalp.

The doctor was carefully clipping away the sun-bleached hair. Then he lathered the remaining close-cropped hair with soap and began to shave Skip's head. Skip felt pulls at his scalp. Then he felt waves of pain as the razor was scraped over and over against his scalp, removing any trace of hair. Even with the pain, Skip tried to visualize what he would look like with no hair.

"Dumb," he thought to himself.

Dr. Neal was leaning over him again.

"Skip, you're going to feel a slight pinch on the right side of your head. It won't last but a second," he said softly.

Skip did feel the pinch. It didn't hurt. It was just as Dr. Neal had said.

There was silence for a time, then Skip thought he heard the whine of a drill behind his head. He felt a slight pressure against his head. Then he was sure he heard the sound of a drill. It was close to him. Right above his right ear.

The sound stopped.

Then he heard it again. This time it was close to his left ear.

He again felt slight pressure against his skull. There was no pain.

Skip was tired. Very tired. He couldn't fully accept the fact that he was lying on a hospital table. He blinked to stay awake.

There was a different sound now. The drilling noise had stopped. Skip could hear, very clearly, a slow crunching sound.

The noise continued. Then stopped.

It started again. Then stopped again.

There was a rhythm to it. A pattern. Someone was turning a screw.

The sound stopped again. It was a longer time before it began again. Skip recognized the same rhythm when it started again.

He was horrified. They were screwing something into his head. He wanted to scream, to leap off the table, to get out. His arms and legs wouldn't move. He was a captive inside his body.

The crunching sound stopped and Dr. Neal looked down at Skip again.

"We're all finished for right now, Skip. You've done just fine. I'll be back in a few minutes. I want to talk to your mother and father," he said.

The quiet that briefly enveloped Skip was broken by the voice of a black man in a white uniform.

"I'm gonna have to cut your bathing suit off you. Won't hurt. You just relax," the orderly said.

Skip thought about the suit. A Hang-Ten. Almost new. "No," he thought. "Why would he want to cut it?"

He managed to speak. "No. It's a new Hang-Ten. You can't cut it. I'll need it later."

The man retreated, pulling the curtain open, then closing it. Skip was beginning to hate the sound of the metal rings sliding across the curtain rod. The sound meant someone was coming to do something to his body or someone was leaving him to be alone with his fear and confusion.

Skip heard the man talking to a nurse outside the curtain.

"He doesn't want it cut off him. What should I do?" the man asked the nurse.

"I'll see what I can do," she replied.

The sound of the curtain opening and closing again.

A nurse smiled down at Skip. "We have to get it off. But maybe we don't have to cut it. Let's try," she said.

The nurse and the black man worked slowly and carefully, easing the suit down and finally off. Skip felt nothing as the two of them moved his arms and legs to remove the suit.

A new doctor came in.

"Skip. Skip, you're doing just fine. We're going to catheterize you now. And then we'll let you get some rest," he said.

The doctor continued, anticipating the question asked by Skip's puzzled and frightened look.

"Skip, you're paralyzed. You can't void. This will help you," he said.

Skip was still confused. He still didn't know what was going to happen. But he didn't ask.

The doctor continued to explain.

"It's a small tube. We are going to insert it into your penis. You won't feel it. I promise you."

Skip surrendered completely to mounting terror. The shaving. The drill. The sound of the screws. Now they were going to put something inside his penis.

He had, until that moment, tried to find the courage and the strength to ask one more question.

Now he was too scared to ask whether he was going to die.

Patsy Wilkins clasped her hands so tightly together that her fingers turned crimson. She sat quietly in the waiting area outside the emergency room of Norfolk General. Some of her fear would disappear when Tommy arrived, but she knew now that her son was badly hurt. She, too, looked for some answer, some clue to what was happening in the events that had brought her to Norfolk General, accompanying her son in an ambulance.

Patsy, Karen and Shirley had seen Skip earlier in the day. She and her two daughters were having lunch in the drugstore of the shopping center where Skip was working part time. He had come in for Cokes and coffee for his fellow workers. She had told him to be careful that afternoon at Lake Joyce where he was going water skiing. He had smiled at her and responded as he always did when she was protective, "Aw, Mom, come on." Then he was gone.

Later that afternoon at home, as she was trying to shake off a bad headache, the phone had rung. It was Yvonne O'Brien, the mother of Skip's friend Gary.

"Patsy," Yvonne said, "Gary just called. There's been an accident with the boat. Skip's been hurt. He's at Virginia Beach Hospital now. You need to go."

Patsy's first thought was about the motorboat.

"Yvonne, he's not cut up, is he?" The ugliness of propellers slicing into her son's body flashed through her mind, but the thought was too dreadful to remain.

"No. No, Patsy. No, he's not cut up."

"Are you sure? 'Cause I have to call Tommy. I don't think I could handle that."

Yvonne reassured her. "No, he's not cut. He's all right, really, just shaken up, I think. But I think you'd better come on down."

Patsy pressed the disconnect button on the phone and dialed the house where her oldest daughter, Linda, was babysitting.

"Linda. It's Mom. Skip's been hurt. I have to go to the hospital. But I need to send the girls over to you."

Linda's voice was calm. "Okay. Now everything's going to be all right. Don't get upset. And be careful driving. He's fine, I'm sure."

Patsy directed Karen and Shirley to the neighbor's house and set out for the hospital in Skip's car. She talked to herself the whole way, reminding herself to stay calm. She was not familiar with his car or the way to the hospital and she made a wrong turn.

When she pulled up to the emergency room entrance, she spotted Gary O'Brien sitting outside. He was crying. Patsy stooped down and put her hands on his shoulders. "Gary," she said, "there's nothing to cry about. You know Skippy's going to be fine."

As soon as Patsy identified herself to the nurse at the counter, she was ushered into the emergency area where starched white curtains were pulled back at the front of each small cubicle. A doctor met her.

"Mrs. Wilkins. Your son is resting comfortably right now. But he's injured his neck. Badly. It may be broken."

Patsy wanted to see her son. She nodded to the doctor and headed toward the one cubicle that was occupied. Nearing the foot of the bed, she recognized him. He was lying still. Only his chest was moving, heaving slightly with his breathing. His arms were folded across his chest, his eyes were closed. His body, what she could see of his shoulders, was deeply tanned from weekends of surfing and being on the beach. There were no marks, no wounds on her son. She went limp with relief.

Skip opened his eyes.

"Skippy, don't you worry. You're going to be fine. God will take care of you. You know that."

She leaned down and gently kissed his cheek. Skip felt a tear form in the corner of his eye, and then roll down the side of his face.

"I hope so, Mom," Skip said in a weak voice. "I sure hope so." He wanted to share her belief right now.

Patsy composed herself before she dialed Tommy's number. She reported to her husband what she had learned, told him where she was and hung up.

A doctor appeared at her side and motioned her toward the semi-privacy of the emergency room and away from the corridor.

"Mrs. Wilkins," he said, "we're going to have to transfer your son to Norfolk General."

"Why?" Patsy asked. "Isn't he all right here? He looks fine. What is . . ."

The doctor broke in. His voice was soft, but urgent.

"Mrs. Wilkins, it does appear that your son has a broken neck. We don't have a neurosurgeon here."

"No. No, wait a minute." Patsy was panicking. "I have to call my husband. Skippy's uncle is a doctor and I want to talk to him. He'll know what to do."

This time the doctor let her finish. Then he spoke. "Mrs. Wilkins, we've just contacted Norfolk General. They are expecting him. And we've talked to the doctors there and they'll be waiting. You can ride with your son, but we really do need to move him as quickly as we can."

Patsy rushed back to the phone. She dialed Tommy's number again to tell him to go to Norfolk General. She was told that he had already left the office. She was frantic, but only for a moment. Skip was being rolled out of the emergency room and toward the door.

Two men in white uniforms of the volunteer rescue squad carefully collapsed and locked the legs of the stretcher-bed and lifted it and its occupant into the back of the ambulance.

Patsy and an attendant sat in the back with Skip.

The ride was uneventful for the first 10 minutes and Patsy began to relax, although she didn't take her eyes off her son's face.

Skip began to vomit. A watery green liquid oozed out of the side of his mouth and ran down his cheek. Before the attendant could move to him, his body began contracting as the lake water and weed particles in his system were regurgitated in waves of green. He began to choke. He gasped for air. He couldn't breathe.

Patsy wanted to scream and get out of the ambulance. But she couldn't take her eyes off Skip.

The attendant reached behind Skip's head and neck with both hands and quickly and carefully turned Skip's head ever so slightly to allow him to empty his mouth and throat and begin to breathe. All the while the attendant talked to him and reassured him.

The attendant leaned toward the small window to the cab and the driver. In a soft and matter-of-fact voice, he said, "He's going into shock. He's into shock, I think."

The attendant worked to keep Skip's throat clear. When the vomiting appeared to end, he cleaned Skip's face and placed an oxygen mask over Skip's mouth and nose.

As soon as the ambulance pulled in front of the emergency room doors, attendants came out and assisted in getting Skip inside.

A doctor told Patsy that they were going to begin taking X-rays and that she should try not to worry, that they would get back to her as soon as they knew something.

Patsy was now desperate for her husband. She was beginning to buckle emotionally. She needed his strong reassurance. Patsy wanted Tommy. She needed him. As the doctors began their examination of Skip, Patsy was left alone to deal with the events of the past two hours. She prayed and talked to God. It helped, but she knew she would be better only when her husband came. She wondered how long it would take. He'd have to go to the Beach hospital first, then retrace part of his journey back into Norfolk. "Hurry. Please hurry, Tommy. I can't hold on much longer," she said to herself.

When Tommy rushed through the doors and she caught sight of him, Patsy was relieved. She felt stronger and suddenly believed that everything would be all right. She told him quickly what she knew and he had disappeared into the emergency room to find his son.

Patsy and Tommy rose from their chairs in the waiting area of the emergency room when they saw Bill Butler coming toward them.

Tears were trickling down his face as he joined them. He was a doctor. But he was also family. And the family part of him was ruling now.

He looked first at Tommy, then at Patsy. He blinked his eyes, then spoke to them.

"You know, I only wish that it were me in there."

"Uncle Bill. Oh, Uncle Bill. Why do you say that?" Patsy asked.

"Because my life is almost over. And his is just beginning. He has so much promise."

He paused a moment. "Patsy, Skip may never walk again." His voice cracked as the words came out. More tears formed in his eyes.

"You need to talk to Dr. Neal. But I thought I ought to tell you that myself."

Dr. Neal joined them.

He recognized the question in their minds by the fright in their eyes. He waited a second to see if they wanted to speak. When they didn't, he gave them the only answer he had.

"It is very, very bad. The very worst. He will probably never walk again."

"No," Patsy said firmly. "He'll walk again. He will walk. Skippy will walk."

Dr. Neal touched her arm.

"You hang onto that faith," he said.

Dr. Neal told them that Skip was being moved to an operating room and then would be put in intensive care. He suggested that they would be more comfortable in the family waiting room on the ICU ward. He left to return to Skip.

When the elevator doors opened on to the ICU floor, Patsy and Tommy saw dozens of people already in the halls and crowding the main waiting room. Friends. Family. Boys who they recognized as Skip's friends.

The knots of people clogging the hallway parted as Tommy and Patsy made their way to the family waiting room. Hands reached out to pat them, heads nodded to them, but no one spoke because no one knew what to say.

The word had spread rapidly about Skip — from Linda to Skip's grandparents, from Gary to Skip's friends. Adults and high school students had stopped what they were doing and driven to the hospital. Nobody really knew for sure what had happened, but all of them knew that it was serious. Some had heard that Skip had died. People continued to come in. Relatives and close family friends came in the family room to speak to Tommy and Patsy, then resumed in their vigils in the hallway.

The waiting came to an end when Dr. Neal appeared.

"Before you go in and see him," he said, "I want you to understand what has happened." He explained that the fourth, fifth and sixth vertebrae of Skip's spine had been crushed.

"Don't be alarmed when you see him. We've shaved his head in order to put him in Crutchfield tongs. They look a little bit like the tongs you'd use to lift a block of ice. They're to keep his neck in traction. He is conscious and you can talk to him for a minute."

Tommy and Patsy followed the doctor.

Neither of them had absorbed what Dr. Neal had told them. Neither of them knew what Crutchfield tongs were. They wanted only to see their son.

When Dr. Neal pulled back the curtain to the ICU cubicle, Tommy and Patsy Wilkins weren't prepared for the sight that was in front of them in the dim light.

Skip's body, naked to the waist, was fully developed and nearly perfect in its proportions. The well-defined muscles glistened from his tan even in the dimness. His was the body of a young athlete.

From his neck upwards, he was a picture of torture. He was bald. Dried blood splotched his forehead where his head had been scraped in the accident. Blood had dried around several cuts suffered when his head was shaved. Tongs, large steel tongs, were clamped into his skull and attached to a cable running to the head of his bed. Blood that had oozed from the drill holes had dried and crusted around the openings in his skull where the tip of the tongs entered. His head was fixed toward the ceiling, held immobile by the hideous tongs.

Patsy and Tommy Wilkins were standing in a horror chamber. Their son was the victim. Each reached instinctively for the other's hand. When they touched, the hands fit together and each of them squeezed hard, trying to make the pain and the awesomeness of what they saw go away.

They both moved to the head of the bed and leaned over so that Skip could see the two of them. They were afraid to touch him. They continued to clasp hands.

Finally Patsy spoke. "Skippy. We're here. You're going to be fine now. The doctors are taking care of you. And God is going to look after you. You hear?''

Tommy leaned close to his son. ''Skip, we're going to be with you. We're going to work this out. You're going to be all right, son.''

Skip's eyes acknowledged that he heard their words.

They stepped back from the bed and slowly walked out of the room and back to the waiting room.

Dr. Neal joined them. ''If you are praying people, now is the time to pray.'' He squeezed each of them on the arm and returned to ICU.

Patsy sat on the sofa. She was quiet and calm for a moment. But then her mother, who had moved next to her, began to sob. The vision of her son with those awful tongs in his head, lying so still on the bed, came back to Patsy. She felt tears flow down her cheeks. She didn't try to stop them or to wipe them away. She gazed at the walls straight ahead, crying.

Tommy had to walk. Anywhere. Down the hall. Anywhere. But he had to walk right now.

Friends nodded as he went past, but none spoke. They all saw the sadness in his face.

When he reached the end of the hall, he found Paul Bradley, one of Skip's friends. As their eyes met, they both wept. They didn't speak, but somehow they both understood that Skip was in terrible trouble.

5

The vigil that began the night of Skip's accident became a routine for Patsy and Tommy.

It was midnight when they left the hospital and went home that first night. Patsy's aunt, Irene Wagner, and her husband — Auntie and Uncle Ackie — were waiting. The two had hurried from their Norfolk home to stay with the three girls as soon as they had heard about Skip. They had wanted to be with Patsy and Tommy at the hospital, but they felt they could better serve the crisis by looking after the children.

Tommy and Patsy gathered everyone in the living room. There, they told them as much as they understood about Skip's accident and what had happened to him.

The girls gave way to tears as soon as they were told that their brother was badly hurt. They idolized Skip. He took care of them. He babysat with them. He teased them. He played with them. He stood up for them and he protected them. He was the local football star, but, more importantly, he was their brother.

Tommy and Patsy comforted their daughters through the tears, fought back their own, and finally went to bed, totally drained.

They slept for three hours, rising before dawn to return to the hospital where they waited for the precious five minutes out of each hour that they were allowed to be with their son.

Tommy and Patsy became constant occupants of the ICU waiting room. When they reminded themselves to eat, they went to the hospital's snack bar. One or the other sometimes would go home for a while to help Linda with the two girls. But that was all they saw of the world outside Norfolk General for the first nine days.

The outside world, however, managed to intrude into their lives behind the hospital walls.

The local newspapers wanted to know about Skip: his accident, how it happened, his condition, his future. It was a normal series of questions. Skip's name, his picture, his athletic records in football and track, and his acceptance of a college football scholarship had been part of the local sports news for the past two years. Now he was injured. The newspaper wanted to tell the readers how and how badly.

In addition, friends of the Wilkins family and Skip's school friends were flooding the hospital switchboard with calls and questions.

The queries led to a discussion among the two Wilkins, the doctors and the hospital administrator.

"We're going to have to release some kind of statement," the administrator said.

Tommy could see no problem. He and his wife were ready to acknowledge to the outside world exactly what they could understand: their son had a broken neck.

That phrase, however, was too blunt for the doctors and the administrator.

The statement, when it was released to the press, read that Skip "is progressing well. He has sustained severe neck injuries and is being treated in the intensive care unit of Norfolk General Hospital."

The news story explained that Skip had been injured when his water skis struck a rock in a shallow section of Lake Joyce in Virginia Beach. It quoted Tommy as saying that his son had been skiing since he was six years old and that his was his first serious accident.

There was no reference in the story to Skip Wilkins' future. That question couldn't be answered, so it wasn't raised in the newspaper.

As a result of the discussion with the doctors and the administrator about the newspaper statement, Tommy began to understand that he knew very little about Skip's condition. He realized that he needed to ask questions of every doctor and every nurse assigned to his son. There were subtleties among medical people that he would never understand unless he began to question and question hard.

One thing that he and Patsy did understand was the ever-present possibility of death during the first days of Skip's hospitalization.

Dr. Neal had explained to them that swelling could set in as a result of the crushed vertebrae. The swelling, throughout Skip's body, would begin slowly and unhaltingly to squeeze off his air supply. This shock to his already weakened system would be followed by death.

If the swelling started, and it was most likely to occur during the first 72 hours after the accident, there was little that anyone could do to reverse the outcome.

Each time Patsy and Tommy saw Dr. Neal during the first days and nights, their immediate comfort in his presence gave way to fear when he started to speak.

But each time, Dr. Neal reported, ''He's holding his own.'' They would feel relief. Then they would find more courage for the next meeting.

They tried not to think about what could happen, but it was there. Minute after waking minute, they lived with the knowledge that their son could begin to die.

Early on the morning of the fourth day, Dr. Neal had a different message. ''He's made it. He's passed this crisis. I don't think that we need to worry about the swelling anymore. I think it would have begun before now. We've been very fortunate.'' He smiled at them. He still had a lot to do for his young patient, but he was aware that the words he had just spoken had given new strength and hope to the Wilkinses.

Tommy and Patsy grabbed at the news, viewing it as a major victory. They wanted to know what the next step would be.

''If he continues to show improvement,'' Dr. Neal said, ''the next move will be out of ICU and into a regular room. He's a remarkable young man. Without his strength and his physical conditioning, I don't think he would have come this far. I know it's hard to see right now, but you are fortunate that he is such a strong young man.''

A move out of ICU became the next prayed-for event in the life of the Wilkins family.

Tommy, without knowing why and without telling anyone, began to keep a diary on Skip in a small pocket-size notebook that he had pulled from his sportcoat the first night in the hospital.

His first entry read:

> ''6-12-67
> ''Injured.
> ''Taken to VB hospital by rescue squad. Taken
> to Norfolk General Hosp. as no neurosurgeon
> avail. He was taken off stretcher and replaced
> on stretcher at VB hospital.
> ''X-rayed at General.
> ''Doctors comment (it is the worst, the future

looks very dim). Put in intensive care unit of
Norfolk Gen.''

On June 19, the eighth day of Skip's stay in ICU, Tommy turned
slowly through the notebook as he waited for the time he could see his
son.

There had been little to note during the previous days.

"6-13-67 (tues.)
"Pain and uncomfortable."

The same entry was made for Wednesday, June 14.
On June 15 and June 16, Tommy had noted:

"Soft diet. Liquids."

The next two days, June 17 and June 18, the notation in the small
book read simply:

"Sick stomach."

Tommy wondered what the eighth day and night, June 19, would
bring to his son.

Skip seemed stronger and more rested when he and Patsy reached
the side of his bed. His stomach was settled and he had been able to hold
down some liquids.

There had been little conversation among the three during the past
days and nights. Skip either had been in pain or had been too exhausted
to talk. Now he wanted to talk.

"You know how you two have been telling me that God will take
care of me, Mom? And Dad, you told me that God will show us the
purpose in all of this. Well, I've been thinking." Skip paused.

He took a deep breath and continued.

"Well, I've made up my mind that I am going to get better. I know
that God will take care of me. And if He does, I'm going to be in college
in the fall. I won't be able to play football, I know. Not this year. But

I'll be strong enough to play next year. And if I work hard enough, I can play pro ball after college. I'm going to do it. I've decided. I'm going to do it as a testimony to God.''

His parents didn't try to discourage him; they had witnessed the first positive sign from their son. There would be time enough later to tell Skip the truth about his condition. When he was stronger and could handle it. They let him continue to talk, easing his mind by agreeing with him that the coach at Elon College, the North Carolina school Skip had decided on, would probably hold his scholarship open until next season.

As Tommy sat again in the waiting room, urging the clock to speed its hands so he could be with his son one more time, he reached for his notebook. Under the date of June 19, 1967, he wrote:

> ''Skip said college next yr. No football. Then
> good at football and pro ball as a testimony to
> God!''

Tommy wanted to believe that it could be done, but he knew better. He had seen the X-rays. Perhaps someday there would be football, but it wouldn't be next year.

Skip, lying quietly in his bed, thought about his decision. Since he was a child, he had never doubted God's existence. He'd been raised to believe. Now, with God as his only hope, he was more than willing to promise that his recovery and a football career would be a testimony to the God that his mother and his father kept so close to them.

Time was measured in victories and defeats, not days and nights. Hope and despair traveled sometimes on the smallest of events.

Skip's only body movement was with his right arm. Frequently he would sense his nose itching. Or the set of prism glasses that allowed him some outward vision began to cause headaches. On those occasions, he would instinctively raise his arm towards his face. With concentration, he could lift it into the air. The muscles remained in deep shock. When his arm neared a vertical position, it became uncontrollable and would fall back as dead weight, frequently smashing down across his face.

He developed serious nose bleeds as his wrist constantly slammed down against his nose. Finally a doctor was summoned to pack his nose. Skip told him that he felt like something was caught in his throat. He couldn't breathe well. The doctor suctioned his throat, clearing the passage of blood that had been continually collecting from his damaged nose.

Skip spent a restless night and had increasing difficulty in taking deep breaths. When the nurse came in for morning rounds, Skip told her that he thought he had something in his throat. First one nurse, then a second examined him. They saw nothing.

Uncle Bill appeared at his bedside as he had done each morning since Skip had been admitted. It was one way that Skip could tell when morning came in the dim, unchanging world of ICU.

"How're you feeling this morning, Skip? Sleep well last night?" he asked his nephew.

"I can't breathe, Uncle Bill. I feel like something's in my throat."

Bill Butler examined his throat.

He became urgent, demanding a spittle. He reached his hand into Skip's mouth, searching the throat with his fingers.

Skip gagged. He thought he was going to vomit. It felt as though his uncle's whole fist was in his throat. Skip felt a sucking sensation, then the sensation of an object moving in his throat. His mouth filled up.

His uncle withdrew his hand and carefully turned Skip's head to one side. Instinctively Skip discharged the contents of his mouth. A large blood clot fell into the spittle.

"This boy could have choked to death," he heard his uncle tell the nurses.

"The next time he says he has something in his throat, there *is* something in his throat. Either get it out yourselves or call a doctor. Let's get a humidifier in here. That will help his breathing."

Bill patted him on the arm and left for his rounds.

Skip's nose and throat became two new concerns for nurses and doctors.

The following day, June 21, brought a victory. Skip was moved from ICU to the C Wing of Norfolk General. Almost daily Tommy or Patsy had asked Dr. Neal when Skip could be moved; it became an obsession with them. Dr. Neal had seen some improvement in his patient, but he believed that the more time Skip's parents could spend with him, the more quickly Skip might regain his spirit and his strength. Dr. Neal now felt that a move from ICU was medically and emotionally wise. Elation showed on Skip's face and on Patsy's as she walked beside her son, being wheeled down the corridors to a hospital room.

The move, when it was completed, was not joyous. C Wing was in the older section of the hospital. New paint would have been welcome and the room was not bright and airy. An older man, who had suffered a broken neck, was in one of the two beds. A woman and a child were visiting in the room when Skip was wheeled in. The patient was smoking. A television set was on, although no one seemed to be watching it.

Patsy was deflated. The atmosphere had been brighter and more pleasant in ICU. Skip, too, had been hit by the sudden depressing change. The move had been built up in both of them as something positive. It wasn't. Patsy made up her mind that Skip would be moved, that day. When Tommy arrived from work, he quickly agreed. They tried to reach Dr. Neal. He was out of town. The nurses wouldn't move Skip without a doctor's authorization.

An unexpected visitor took Skip's mind away from the depression of his surroundings. His football coach, John Grady, had come to see him. He had brought someone with him. The coach and Skip exchanged greetings.

"Skip, this is Johnny Cooke."

Skip looked up. Bending over him was a young man, tanned and athletic looking. He was smiling down pleasantly at Skip.

"Hi, Skip. Glad to meet you. Coach Grady has told me about you. And about the accident.

"I've got something I want to tell you, something that happened to me not long ago."

Their eyes met for a moment.

"Skip, I broke my neck, too. It happened when I was in college."

Skip's eyes widened. The phrase again. Broken neck. This time the words were coming from a friend, someone Coach Grady had brought. And he was walking.

"You did?"

"Yeah, I sure did. And I had a thing on my head similar to yours. It was more like a chin strap with leather around the top. But it had a weight that held my head in place, just like yours."

"You're kidding. You couldn't have."

"I did. It was 18 days before I could feel anything. Or even move my arm. Then I started to get some return. Now I'm fully recovered."

Skip looked at him. The visitor wasn't kidding. He was standing right there, beside the bed. No wheelchair. No crutches. Standing. His words were the most encouraging words that Skip had heard.

The two men stayed for a brief time. As they said their goodbyes, Skip looked at Johnny Cooke again.

"If he got better in 18 days," Skip thought to himself, "I'm going to be all right in 18 days, too." He made a note of the date, June 21. In 18 days, it would be July 9. "That's the date," Skip told himself, "that I'm going to get well."

Skip had already been persuading himself that he would get well as soon as the tongs were removed. "After all," he thought, "that's what is holding my head straight so my neck can heal." He had another reason for wanting the tongs out. He had seen them in a mirror that his mother had held over him. The tongs were hideous and they made him look sick and ugly and he knew that people didn't want to look at him with those things screwed into his head.

So now he had two goals. First, get the tongs out. Then get through the 18 days, the same time it took Johnny to get better and get out of bed.

Patsy's determination to have her son moved to another room was fueled further after Coach Grady and Johnny Cooke left. A class of student nurses came into the room. They were learning about the care of paralysis cases. Their immediate lesson was the proper use of suppositories on paralysis patients. Skip was to be the patient. Many of the nurses were no older than Skip. Patsy controlled her anger, but flatly told the senior nurse that Skip would not be used in such a lesson. She added that episode to her reasons to get Skip to a different room.

She was adamant about the move. She pulled a chair closer to Skip's bed and made herself comfortable. She had made up her mind that she was going to stay with her son until he was moved.

Visiting hours had been over for nearly an hour when a nurse came in. "Mrs. Wilkins, I'm afraid you'll have to leave now. We'll take good care of him until the morning."

"I'm not leaving, nurse, until he's out of this room." Patsy's voice was a near-whisper because of the sleeping patients, but it conveyed determination.

The nurse withdrew and returned minutes later with the floor nurse.

"Mrs. Wilkins," the senior nurse said, "we do have to ask you to leave. Your son will be all right. We'll . . ."

Patsy cut her off.

"I'm not leaving. Not until he's moved. You can get anybody else you want to tell me to leave. But I'm not going. Period. Not until he's out of this wretched room."

The nurses retreated together. The next time one of them came into the room, nothing was said about leaving. Patsy had made her point.

During the night Skip had been turned slightly to one side by the nurses and he saw his fellow patient. The man's leg, lifeless from paralysis, was dangling out of the bedsheets at an awkward and painful looking angle. The sight struck Skip with terror. The man suffered the same spinal damage as Skip. If the man had no feeling in his leg, then Skip couldn't feel anything in his own limb. He was looking at his own condition.

For the first time, Skip acknowledged that he was paralyzed. He thought back to ICU, the near darkness and the blips and beeps of the machines, the hushed tones of the nurses and the soft rolling of a bed out of ICU when a patient died and was removed from those who still had some life left.

Visions of the past days rushed at him: his father leaning over him, telling him that his neck was broken; his confusion when he tried, without anyone's urging or anyone's presence, to move his legs and felt nothing, not sure whether they had moved because he couldn't lift his head to see his legs; the awful fear of dying after the doctor drilled into his head and put the catheter in him; the blacking out after the catheter from fright and exhaustion; the waking later in confusion, having blotted from his mind all of the horror he had experienced. Now those events came back, overwhelming him and frightening him.

He couldn't take his eyes off the leg dangling awkwardly from the bed next to him.

Patsy came to his bedside to check on him.

Only then was Skip able to force his eyes away from the reminder that he, too, was helpless and paralyzed. He looked up at his mother and pleaded softly.

"Mom, don't leave. Please don't leave me. I'm scared."

Patsy pulled the chair closer to his bed for the night.

The next morning Patsy and Tommy continued their pressure to have Skip moved. They had a discussion with Dr. Neal, who had come back on duty. He did not feel that Skip had to be moved.

"I don't care. I want him moved. Out of this room," Patsy interrupted, her voice trembling with anger.

Dr. Neal needed these two people on his side. Skip's battle was going to be tough enough without a feud between his parents and his doctor over a room. Dr. Neal deferred and Skip was moved. A sense of victory returned to Skip and his parents. He was out of ICU and was going into better surroundings, Room 647 in the A Wing.

Within hours of his transfer, baskets of fruit began to arrive. The next day several cards came in the mail. The grapevine was at work again. His relatives, advised of the transfer out of ICU, passed the information to Skip's friends. A recreation center, close to Skip's home, raised enough money to buy him a television set.

Skip's spirits began to climb, but most of his body remained limp and lifeless. His chart, had he been allowed to see it, would have sucked out his remaining strength and fight. "Quadriplegia below the C-6 dermatomal level. He has anesthesia below the C-6 level . . . The function of his triceps muscles, finger flexors, intrinsic hand muscles, intercostal and legs is absent."

There were days when the medical staff thought there might be some response in his legs, only to find a day later that it had disappeared. Tommy recorded each incident in his notebook, his own spirits rising and falling with the content of each cryptic phrase.

Twelve days after the accident, Skip managed another victory. His stomach had rebelled at almost every solid that he had been fed. His relatives had begun to bring all kinds of food to him, hoping to discover something that his system would not reject. His uncle, Eddie Hutcheson, had brought a handful of grapes one afternoon and tenatively fed them to his nephew. Skip enjoyed them and they stayed down. Shortly after that discovery, Tommy had begun to place a single grape in his open palm and to encourage Skip to try to pick it up and eat it. The exercise was agonizing. Skip had so little use of his fingers that he was unable to hold a grape, but he kept trying. Hour upon hour and day following day of patience and effort finally brought results. He was able to grasp a grape between the knuckle of his thumb and his index finger without crushing it or dropping it.

He had lost so much ability in his arm that the limb would still collapse when he lifted it into the air. His hand, still holding the grape, would fall across his face, sometimes reinjuring his nose, other times bruising his mouth or chin. It was on a Saturday, as Tommy held the grape in his hand and encouraged his son to pick it up, that Skip managed to get a single grape into his mouth.

He had fed himself.

It was a single grape, but it also was another sign of progress for father and son. That night Tommy entered the feat in his well-thumbed notebook.

There was no sign of the use of muscles or nerves returning, however. The doctors and nurses rotated the checks they made over his body. One day they worked with his fingers, the next his arms, then his legs. Occasionally there was a sudden movement in a limb. Once both legs appeared to respond to a stimulus in one leg. But the doctors patiently explained away Tommy's hope for his son's recovery. They explained that muscle spasms occurred, even in cases of paralysis.

Skip was aware only that he was making progress. He didn't ask for details. He didn't want to know anything except when he would get well. So he didn't ask. And neither his parents nor his doctors volunteered anything except encouragement and frequent compliments about his cooperation with the ceaseless picking and probing at his body.

He found increasing comfort and enjoyment in the stream of friends and acquaintances who came to visit. Each person's appearance at the door to his room brought a genuine smile to his face. Some were timid in coming into the room; some were awkward in trying to find something to say, but Skip was relaxed with all of his visitors and they quickly relaxed in his presence. He kidded with his friends and joked about his appearance. He was losing weight, his suntan had faded and his hair, beginning to grow out again, was too long to lie flat and too short to respond to a comb or brush.

He felt a sense of obligation to everyone who expressed his concern about him. Almost daily, there was some new acknowledgement of his courage. Local radio stations periodically mentioned him and asked listeners to send cards and offer prayers of recovery for him. A group of friends organized a benefit dance to raise funds for his family. His entire recreation league softball team, all in uniform, came to see him before one of their games.

Harvey Shapiro had called and wanted to come by to visit. Skip was puzzled. Why would Harvey come by? They had gone to junior high together, but Harvey had been injured in a diving accident in the ninth grade and Skip had seen him only once since then — sitting in a wheelchair at a party.

As Skip was still pondering the questions, there was a knock on the door.

In moments, the smiling face of Harvey Shapiro was in Skip's full view. Skip remembered now that Harvey had been small. He hadn't grown in the three years since junior high. He seemed even smaller now, swallowed up in his wheelchair. Harvey's father spoke to Skip and took a seat by the window.

As the two boys chatted about the few mutual friends that they still shared, Skip began to wonder how Harvey had dealt with his accident. The living in a wheelchair. "How," Skip wondered, "could Harvey smile and laugh and seem so content after all he'd been through and what he had to look forward to. Three years in a wheelchair and he'd probably never get out of it."

Harvey began telling Skip of his experiences. Soon Skip was hearing some of the same words and terms that he heard from his own doctors.

As Harvey talked, he spoke of people's reaction to a crippled individual, how his mind wasn't crippled and how some people were able to accept him as a person in spite of the wheelchair. He told Skip about his ability to go places, with the help of the attendant his family had found. He said that he was able to have fun with other young people, even drink and go to parties.

The longer Harvey talked, the more Skip wished that he would go away. Skip knew that he was different. He was going to get well. Johnny Cooke had gotten well, hadn't he?

Harvey and his father finally left. Skip was relieved, but the things that Harvey had told him stuck in his mind. He tried to tell himself that he was going to get well, just like Johnny Cooke. It was only days away. How many? He tried to do the mental arithmetic, but Harvey's story kept getting in the way.

Finally Skip thought he understood why Harvey Shapiro had come to see him. He had come to help, to tell Skip what lay ahead, to help him realize that he was in for disappointments, but that life for a cripple wasn't all bad.

Skip tried to reject the possibility, but the vision of Johnny Cooke, standing tall and straight and healthy beside his bed kept fading away. In its place was the picture of Harvey Shapiro in a wheelchair.

It was the last time that Skip would put all of his hope in Johnny Cooke's visit and it was the last time that he would secretly count the days — the 18 magic days — until he got well.

Somewhere between what had happened to Johnny Cooke and what was never going to happen to Harvey Shapiro was the answer for Skip Wilkins.

Despite his apprehensions about the future that came more frequently, Skip worked hard to be positive and cheerful with those around him, especially his parents.

There were times, though, especially at night when he was alone, that a sense of hopelessness would overcome him. In those moments, which he kept secret even from his parents, he always managed to rally, to look ahead and to find hope by remembering the scores of people who cared about him and who kept him in their thoughts and prayers.

Skip's improving spirits and his interest in his visitors provided an opportunity for Tommy and Patsy to survey their worlds outside the hospital's walls and to turn their attentions for a while to their other responsibilities.

Tommy concentrated with renewed dedication on his job. He had stayed at the hospital for nine days and there was plenty of work to be caught up. When he returned to the office, his boss called for him.

"Tommy," he said, "I want you to know that we're all pulling for Skip. We know that he's going to make it through this thing all right. If we can help at all, just let us know. I know it's tough right now and I know that you want to be with him as much as you can. We'll work together with you. And if you have to be with him on short notice, just let us know."

It was this attitude at work and the knowledge that he was highly regarded and that everyone was concerned about his son that kept Tommy going at his desk. In his own way, he felt a sense of obligation to the people who cared about him and his son.

Patsy found that she could slip away from Skip without worry when he was expecting visitors. She turned her attention to Linda, who had been managing the house and the chores, and taking care of Karen and Shirley.

Patsy was proud of her daughters. Since the afternoon when she had called her daughter Linda to tell her that Skip had been hurt, Patsy had left the house and the two little girls to Linda's care. There had been no problems.

Linda, 16 and two years younger than Skip, had admired her brother as long as she could remember. She had wanted to become a football player in grammar school because he was one. She had followed his athletics at every home game since his junior high years. They double-dated. She had never resented being "Skip's kid sister" although she had just ended an active year as a high school sophomore. She was worried about Skip, but she had found it natural to assume responsibilty when her parents' lives suddenly were shifted into a hospital.

She drove her sisters every morning to Bible School, returned home and cleaned, picked up the girls, fixed lunches and suppers, and took them to playgrounds, to the beach, to visit their friends and on some weekends, the three of them went to stay with Auntie and Uncle Ackie.

Linda managed to keep up her friendships with her schoolmates and she continued, when she could arrange it with her grandparents as chaperones, to have friends over to visit.

She had been raised as a member of a close and loving family. She was doing what was natural to her.

Only rarely did she overlook the things she knew her mother would want her to do. That was only at mealtime. She and the girls loved pancakes. So pancakes were on almost every breakfast menu, just as hamburgers and french fries were served more than anything else at lunch and at supper.

Only rarely did she let her mind slip into sadness when she thought of her brother lying in the hospital. Sometimes, when she and her sisters and their grandparents would say prayers before bedtime, she would feel tears in her tightly shut eyes. And though she would squeeze her eyes shut even harder, the tears would still come.

Linda had a constant companion to help her around the house. Martha Chevalier was one of Linda's schoolmates and the girl whom Skip had been dating most often during the spring before school had ended. Martha had come to the house as soon as she heard about Skip's accident. From that first night, she was there whenever she could be. She helped Linda with the dishes and with the cleaning. She rode with her on the trips to Bible School. Sometimes she was just there to talk. Linda began to realize that Martha cared very deeply about Skip. And she wondered whether Skip knew that and whether he felt the same way.

Mike Whitley was always around to help the girls, too. He was a friend of Linda and Skip, although Skip was closer to Wayne, the older brother. Mike, without being asked, took over all of the outdoor chores — cutting the grass, trimming the shrubs and keeping the yard neat.

And, sometimes in the background and sometimes in the center of things were Patsy's parents, Granny and Papa, and Auntie and Uncle Ackie.

Whenever Linda and her sisters needed help, someone from the family was there to lend a hand. Someone other than their parents, who couldn't be with them very often. Someone other than their brother, who couldn't be with them at all.

6

The date was June 30 — 18 days since Skip had been admitted to the hospital.

Dr. Neal asked Tommy and Patsy to meet him in the doctor's lounge. Tommy had learned that such a request meant a formal discussion about Skip. Perhaps some new development in his condition. Tommy was uneasy as he and Patsy walked toward the lounge.

"The time has come," Dr. Neal began as they sat down, "to make plans to move Skip."

He didn't wait for a response or a question from either of them. He continued.

"We have done nearly everything that we can do here. He's out of danger as far as shock and as far as further damage is concerned. But we can't do much more to help him gain further use of his remaining nerves and muscles. Assuming there is no unexpected setback, we should be able to remove the tongs in the next week or two. But Skip will need intensive rehabilitation and therapy. There are no facilities available in this area for that kind of treatment."

"Okay. What do you recommend for him? And what should I begin to do?" Tommy was accustomed to his role as the questioner.

The world of doctors, with their unfamiliar terminology, had at first frustrated and intimidated him. He had started asking questions, writing down and remembering terms, learning degrees of physical disability by medical classifications. It had saved him from the feeling of being unable to help his son. He found most of the doctors and nurses helpful and understanding. He began to realize that even they, with all of their knowledge and all of their experience, did not always have absolute answers. In some cases, they had no answers that he wanted to hear.

He had learned a lot about Norfolk General. Now, with Dr. Neal as his tutor, he was about to learn about a different kind of institution.

"There is a place in New York, Tommy. Rusk Institute. It's recognized as one of the leading rehabilitation clinics in the world for the kind of injury that Skip has. I am having my office gather together some information. I am suggesting that we begin now to try to get Skip in there very soon."

"Fine," Tommy said. "Just let me know what I need to do."

Patsy couldn't say anything. She was trying to sort out what she had just heard. She had never given any thought to Skip going anywhere except home.

Tommy sensed her attitude.

"Patsy, we don't have to worry. Skip's making progress, I know. But if Dr. Neal says that he needs to go to a special institute to get even better, then that's what we've got to do. No matter where he goes, we'll be able to see him and it'll be just that much sooner that he can come home for good."

Patsy nodded and tried to shake the feeling of separation from her son that had already set in.

"I know," she said. "I know. It's just that I think he needs us to be with him. To make sure that he's taken care of."

"We'll always make sure of that. But we've got to do what the doctors think is best," Tommy said, helping her up and ending the conversation.

When Tommy arrived at the hospital the next day at lunch, he found his son groggy and tired. Skip had undergone routine and periodic kidney and blood tests. More X-rays had been taken. Skip was complaining of a slight ache in his left shoulder. Dr. Neal had examined the shoulder several days earlier. The shoulder was on the left side, the side that had received the more severe damage. Skip had been told that the slight pain he felt was normal.

Tommy began to act on the information that Dr. Neal's office had provided on Rusk Institute. He quickly hit an obstacle. He was told that Rusk had no available beds and that the institution could not take Skip for several months. He told Patsy, then counseled with Dr. Neal. The next best option was Woodrow Wilson Rehabilitation Center in Fishersville, Virginia. Patsy was relieved when she learned that it was only five hours from home. Tommy began his efforts anew.

Skip began to have frequent headaches. His shoulder remained sensitive. When Tommy visited one Friday morning, Skip complained of chills.

Tommy made a mental note to put an entry in his small diary later and began to help Skip eat some watermelon that had been brought to him. An hour later, the nurse brought lunch. Skip managed to down two bites, then he vomited. Tommy, sensitive to his son's every movement and every act, became convinced that something was going wrong.

Tommy's conviction turned into a reality for Skip. He began to run a low fever and his stomach rejected nearly everything. He began to lose his smile and his optimism. From time to time, he yielded to tears.

Dr. Neal ordered kidney tests for Skip. The tests revealed an infection, but Dr. Neal and a urologist he had called in were relieved. At least they knew where the problem was. Dr. Neal told Tommy and Patsy that at this point, it didn't appear to be too serious.

Skip's face showed relief when he was told that a kidney infection was causing his sickness. He had worried that something was going wrong with his spine and that he was going to suffer even more damage. His spirits were temporarily bolstered, too, when Dr. Neal told him that he was continuing to make progress despite the kidney problem.

Skip used the opportunity to urge that the tongs be taken out. Their removal remained an obsession with Skip, but Dr. Neal declined again to remove them.

"You're not quite ready for that, Skip. But it shouldn't be much longer. We'll see about them when I get back," Dr. Neal said before he left for several days off at nearby Nags Head, North Carolina.

The fact that Dr. Neal also had said that Skip would be going to some kind of rehabilitation place wasn't much consolation and didn't have much impact. It seemed too far away really to grasp and, besides, nothing good was going to happen until the tongs came out. Skip was convinced of that.

The medication prescribed for the kidney infection began to do its work quickly. Skip's fever continued, but his spirit returned and his smile came back.

———

"Good morning, Skip. How're you doing today?"

There was something extra in Dr. Thomson's usual morning greeting, Skip thought to himself. James L. Thomson had taken charge of Skip's case while Dr. Neal was away on vacation.

"Pretty good," Skip said. "Watcha gonna do to me today?"

"Oh, I don't know. Maybe something special. You've been a pretty good patient since Dr. Neal's been gone." Dr. Thomson was leaning over Skip, looking at the patient's head.

Two nurses joined Dr. Thomson. The three of them, a nurse standing on each side of the bed, began working with the weight attached to the tongs. Skip could feel the movement, but he couldn't see what they were doing. He tried to detect what was happening from their soft and infrequent conversation, but he couldn't. He waited and wondered.

Dr. Thomson was again leaning over Skip's head.

Skip thought that the doctor was adjusting the tongs. Someone always seemed to be adjusting them.

Skip felt a slight pressure on one side of his head. He heard a small popping noise as his head was gently jerked to one side.

Suddenly Skip was frightened. He could feel his head rolling from side to side. He tried to stop it, but it wouldn't obey.

"Try to relax, Skip. I know you feel funny. I've just taken the tongs out. They're gone for good."

Dr. Thomson's words didn't help. Skip's head was still rolling from side to side. This wasn't the way it was supposed to be. He was supposed to be better when the tongs came out. But he wasn't. He was worse.

"Put them back," Skip pleaded. "Put them back. I'm going to hurt my neck again."

"Okay, Skip. Just take it easy. Feels funny, I know. But you're fine. Doin' just fine. What you're experiencing is the lack of strong muscles in your neck. We've taken the tongs out and you don't have any support right now. Some of those muscles will come back pretty quickly and you'll be able to control your head. Don't you worry. I wouldn't let you out of here with your head wobbling all over the place. I have to think of my reputation."

Dr. Thomson grasped Skip's shoulder and squeezed it. He looked down at his patient with admiration. Skip managed to smile back.

Skip was exuberant when his parents arrived. He made no effort to suppress his happiness. To the three of them, but especially to Skip, the tongs had represented everything horrible about his injury. They were always there, an extension of his body, an ugly growth coming out of his head, a reminder that his injury was serious, so serious that doctors had to screw things into his skull and place tongs in his head.

The three were joyous. Tommy and Patsy kept asking Skip how it felt to be able to move his head, they kept telling him how well he looked, how normal and how strong he appeared without the tongs. Skip, after the first confusing hour without the ability to control the movement of his head, now experienced the pleasure of being able to turn slowly from side to side and see items in the room that he had only been able to view through the prism glasses or when someone had brought them within his narrow, and always upward, range of vision. The ability to turn his head was so basic, so simple. Yet he had been deprived of that ability for 38 days. Now he delighted in each slight turn, each new angle and the ability to see in all directions.

Just as the dream of an 18-day recovery, like Johnny Cooke's, had faded against the reality of what doctors and medicine could and could not do, so did the healing power that Skip had conjured for the tongs. They were out now and he wasn't well. But he was better and that's what really mattered.

That night at home, Tommy got his notebook from his pocket. He printed in the largest hand that he had used to make his daily entries. The two words told of the biggest victory so far for the three of them:

"7-19-67 TONGS OUT!"

The victory over the tongs was followed by a series of defeats. Skip's fever persisted and Dr. Neal was still out of town.

Tommy and Patsy became impatient with the treatment to reduce the fever. They pressured one of Dr. Neal's associates to do something more about the fever. He responded patiently that he was doing all that he could. Patsy remained concerned.

"With all he's been through, it would seem to me that you would be able at least to get rid of the fever," she told him.

The doctor leveled his eyes on hers.

"Look, Mrs. Wilkins. Your son's spinal cord has been destroyed. He will never walk again. You need to understand that. We will take care of the fever. But don't think for a minute that when the fever's gone that your son is going to get up and walk out of here."

The words seared. No one, not even Dr. Neal, had said that Skip would *never* walk again. She knew the realization of that had stayed hidden deep in her mind. It had come to her on the first night when Dr. Neal had told them, "It is the worst, he may never walk again." But from that moment on, she had pushed that thought out of her consciousness. She wouldn't allow it. There wasn't room. Her thoughts were always on Skip's recovery, on the time when he would come home and start to live his life normally again. That night, for the first time, because of her harsh words about a fever, the thought that her son might never walk again returned to Patsy. This time she had to fight to force it out of her mind.

The fever began to break and the kidney infection began to clear with a change in medication and a change in the type of voiding apparatus that Skip used.

As the kidneys began to clear, another complication developed. Skip's left thigh began to swell and redden. Dr. Neal had returned. His examination indicated a blood clot. He called in a specialist. Skip's leg was elevated and an Ace bandage was carefully wrapped around the thigh. Skip wasn't told how serious the situation was. But Tommy and Patsy were both cautioned to insure that great care was taken with the leg. If the clot moved into his lung, it could mean disaster.

The inflamed leg halted Skip's introduction to a wheelchair. Several days after the tongs had been removed and after he had been measured for a collar and a brace, Skip had been lifted from his bed and placed in a wheelchair. Within minutes he had blacked out. The nurses had expected his reaction and caught him before he slumped and injured himself. Only the four-poster brace kept his head from nodding. The brace fit over his shoulders and had two support bars, one under his chin and the other at the base of the back of his head. He regained consciousness and tried to sit again. Within minutes, he vomited. His first lesson ended.

He became nauseated several more times before he was able to sit for 20 minutes, then 30, then a full hour. Until his leg problem, he had been able to sit for an hour or longer, experiencing only slight dizziness before he was lifted back to bed.

Skip wore a snugly fitting foam collar around his neck, called a Thomas collar, when he was in bed. The collar was replaced with the brace before he was lifted into the wheelchair for periods of sitting.

As Skip worked to build the strength needed to sit for longer and longer periods in a wheelchair, Tommy worked on the arrangements for Skip to go to Woodrow Wilson Rehabilitation Center.

After Dr. Neal's first mention of the center, Tommy had investigated it with the help of Leonard Strelitz, a long-time family friend. It was located 200 miles away in the small town of Fishersville, not far from Waynesboro and Charlottesville. The state had established it in 1947, converting a former Army hospital on the site into the nation's first state-owned and state-operated rehabilitation center.

Tommy had been told that the buildings in use were old, left over from the World War II years, but the state had started work on six new buildings. A couple were already occupied. It had a good reputation, despite the age of the facilities. He'd been told by several doctors and some friends who had checked on the center that it offered some of the best rehabilitation services in the country for the severely handicapped.

He didn't much care about the looks of the place, as long as it offered some hope that his son could get additional help.

Skip's leg problem subsided and he was soon able to sit for long periods in a wheelchair. With the help of nurses and orderlies, he began to visit other patients in the hospital. Most of them knew from the hospital staff about Skip and his injury. He and his family had become favorites among the doctors, nurses, aides and orderlies, many of whom frequented his room when they had time to chat with him or offer him an encouraging word.

On August 9, 1967, nearly two months after Skip had been admitted to Norfolk General Hospital, his father entered a message in his notebook. It read:

"Good Day. Maybe Woodrow Wilson next week."

For the next eight days, the small, informal diary of Tommy Wilkins read the same:

"Good Day."

Nurses from ICU, from the C Wing, and from the A Wing gathered outside the emergency room entrance. Orderlies formed another small congregation. Several doctors were present. All had been touched by Skip's determination. Dozens of other people, young and old, carefully dressed and casually dressed, all friends of Skip, milled outside the entrance. They had assembled to say goodbye.

Skip had no indication of the magnitude of the farewell as his stretcher was rolled outside the emergency room entrance. When he appeared, flanked by his parents, the nurses, orderlies and the group of friends and relatives burst into spontaneous cheers and applause.

Tommy and Patsy were taken aback, too. They had known that several of Skip's friends would be on hand to wish him good luck on his new journey. They hadn't expected members of the hospital staff.

It was a happy occasion for Skip. He managed to say only a couple of sentences before becoming emotional. He thanked the nurses, the orderlies and the doctors for their care and for their interest in him.

He thanked his friends for their concern and for their prayers.

Lastly, just before he was lifted into the ambulance, he thanked his parents and his family for everything that they had done. He acknowledged the sacrifices that they had made to be with him during his stay. He thanked Linda for her watchfulness over his younger sisters and for her care of the house. He wanted everyone to know how wonderful his family was.

Two rescue squadsmen gently lifted the stretcher and placed Skip in the ambulance. Patsy and Tommy climbed into the back with Skip and made themselves as comfortable as they could for the trip. His grandparents walked to their automobile for their drive behind the ambulance.

As the crowd of people, dominated by the white uniforms of nurses and orderlies, waved and shouted their goodbyes to Skip, the ambulance started slowly toward Fishersville, Virginia, and the Woodrow Wilson Rehabilitation Center.

Left behind in the warmth of the August sunshine were almost 50 people who had been touched by Skip's strength and his family's determination to see him well and whole again.

Left behind, as the ambulance pulled out of the driveway and turned onto the street, were hundreds of other people in Tidewater Virginia who had prayed for Skip's recovery and who would the next day be touched when they read in the newspapers that Skip Wilkins, high school athlete, had become strong enough to leave Norfolk General Hospital.

Left behind also were the healing hands of Richard K. Neal, M.D., who that morning had placed a single typewritten page of concise and emotionless medical language inside the stainless steel covers of the case history of Alfred T. Wilkins Jr., 17-year-old white male:

"Discharge Summary
"Re: Alfred T. Wilkins Jr.
"Admitted June 12, 1967
"Discharged August 18, 1967
"The patient, a seventeen-year-old white male
was hospitalized here on June 12, 1967, following a neck injury. Refer to my letter of
July 14, 1967, to Mr. John Wade for details
concerning his injury and early post-injury
course.
"He continued to have an uneventful post-
injury course. The Crutchfield tongs were removed after six weeks of skeletal traction with
satisfactory alignment of the fracture site being
maintained throughout his hospital stay. He
was subsequently increased in his activities
being sent down to daily physiotherapy and
being gotten up in a wheelchair. He has worn
a Thomas collar while in bed and a four-poster
brace when up. He has continued to have satisfactory alignment of the fracture site.
"In early August he developed a complication
thrombophlebitis of his left calf which was
treated with conservative measures including
elevation and wrapping of his legs. The thrombophlebitis cleared without difficulty with the
patient now having only a slight amount of re-

sidual swelling of the left calf region. He developed urinary infections at various times and
was treated with Mandelamine being followed
by the urologist, Doctors Devine, while hospitalized here.

"He is to be transferred today to the Woodrow
Wilson Rehabilitation Center for further care and
treatment. The neurological examination continues to reveal an almost complete quadriplegia
below the C-6 dermatomal level. He is able to
use his biceps muscles and to dorsiflex the wrist
but has only slight function of the finger flexors
and no effective triceps function. He has a complete paralysis of his legs. He has some gross
sensory perception over the legs.

"In conclusion the patient has a transverse
myelopathy with quadriplegia below the C-6 dermatomal level secondary to a compression fracture of the C-5 vertebral body. He has tolerated
his period of skeletal traction and stabilization of
the fracture site without difficulty and is transferred to receive further
rehabilitation."

Richard K. Neal Jr., M.D.

Not left behind on that warm August day were the memories, sometimes hazed by pain, by fear and by lapses into unconsciousness, that
Skip Wilkins alone possessed of his 67-day fight to keep on living.

7

Skip's eyes were fixed on the scenes outside the ambulance as the driver maneuvered along the city streets to reach the highway leading to Fishersville. Through the window across from his stretcher, just to the left of his parents and over his dad's shoulder, he caught sight of car tops, trucks and buses, storefront signs and buildings, and, once in a while, a person. He was out in the real world again. From the window in the hospital everything had seemed distant and remote, untouchable and unreal. Now he could sense the presence of other people and objects that had once been commonplace. He savored the feeling of being alive.

As the ambulance reached the open highway and picked up speed, he shifted his gaze to his body stretched down in front of him, covered by a sheet and a blanket. He took stock of his physique so often now that the sense of sadness and embarrassment were only momentary. He had lost one-third of his body weight during his hospitalization, and was down to 120 pounds. Most of the weight loss had come from his upper body. His chest, once thick and well proportioned, was only loose skin stretched across his rib cage. His arms were nearly bone thin. His biceps and triceps, developed during weeks and weeks of regimented exercise, had softened, then wasted off as he shed his weight.

He knew that he looked unattractive. The emaciated body, the gaunt face with the eyes deep sunk, the short, stubby hair was all that had been left of the handsome, strong athlete of two months ago.

He shifted his eyes to his parents who were talking quietly to each other. Skip studied them for a moment, then eased his head back to its normal straight position, and closed his eyes. He thought how much his parents had done for him during his life, how much love and caring they had given to him and to his sisters, and how much patience they had needed to raise him. He remembered so many incidents and had been told so many others about his strong will and his independence, even as an infant.

With the swaying of the ambulance headed along the highway, Skip lapsed into a reverie.

His mind drifted to North Carolina where the family had bought a small lot on Currituck Sound. It was there that he had begun to learn how close and loving his family was. When he was 11, they worked together, sharing the tasks to clear the land for a trailer. Skip worked next to his father, experiencing the joy of working with his hands, of doing a job — any job — well, and coming to know that work was a proper part of life. He had come to love being on the Sound in the family's small open runabout. More than anything, he liked to be alone in the boat. He would cruise slowly into the Sound, and as soon as he had rounded the point and was out of sight, he would push the throttle wide open and experience the thrill of speed, a thrill that he'd first known when his dad drove the boat. Such trips, Skip remembered, ended with his father's shrill whistle, his index and little finger in each corner of his mouth, and the other hand above his head emphatically motioning for Skip to return to the landing. Once the boat was secured to the landing, he would receive a sharp-tongued lecture or restriction to the trailer, depending on how many times during that summer he had violated the rule against running the boat wide open. He was many years older when he finally understood how his father on the shore, could tell when he, around the point and out of sight, opened the throttle. By then, however, he was old enough to be allowed to handle the boat. His discovery of variable pitch was too late to prevent punishment.

He remembered the woods near his house that had been his special place from the time that he was six years old. No punishment seemed strong enough to keep him in his backyard where his father had built a sandbox and swings and had cleared a large area for marble shooting and later had put up a basketball backboard. He loved the freedom of the woods.

Skip's mind drifted to his early years in school and church. He was frequently ordered to the principal's office. At recess the energy that had built up in him in class became his driving force as he darted around the playground, snatching hats or scarves from the girls and roughhousing with the boys.

It seemed to him that he had gone to Sunday School and to church with his parents as far back as he could remember. Sometimes he skipped Sunday School and went to the store near the church, buying candy with his offering money. Occasionally his teacher would discover his truancy and report it to his parents. On other occasions, after he had returned to the church grounds, the guilt would rise up and he would begin to fear that God was going to punish him. On such occasions, he would promise himself not to do it ever again, but the temptation the next time was greater than the recollection of his fright at God's possible wrath.

Skip's thoughts were interrupted by the slowing of the ambulance, its turn off the highway, and a smooth stop.

"Skip," his father said. "We're stopping here for gas. Do you want a Coke or anything?"

"Ah . . . a Coke," Skip answered.

His father smiled and patted Skip's shoulder as he stooped to make his way to the door.

Skip watched through the open door as his father headed toward the filling station. Skip thought about the times that he and his father had been together and how much his father had taught him. They had worked together when Skip was 9 or 10 to close in the breezeway of their home to make a den. He remembered the tongue-lashings when he'd day-dream on the job and fail to respond to his father's instructions. His father could become very angry, but somehow he always meted out the punishment in a way that left Skip still feeling wanted and loved.

Of all the people Skip knew and admired, his dad was the one person Skip wanted most of all never to disappoint.

There had been disappointments. The keenest ones, the ones that Skip most remembered, had come in athletics. It was there that father and son had a special bond and shared a special pride.

Skip's first athletic competition came in the third grade when he had been selected to represent his class in a track meet. He took instantly to athletics, although he had to work harder than most children to do well.

He had gained a starting position on the community league basket-ball team in the seventh grade. He practiced longer and harder than the others, often working out with his dad in the backyard. He was the top scorer and the team leader going into the last half of the season.

His dad had cautioned him that athletics was only one part of grow-ing up, that schoolwork was equally important. Skip always nodded his understanding after such talks, but he couldn't find a way to enjoy homework and studying. Besides, his parents had always told him that they would be satisfied with Cs on his report cards.

As the end of basketball season approached, Skip turned all of his attention to the game. Twice his dad reminded him of poor grades and twice his dad said that Skip had to improve his report card if he wanted to stay on the team. Skip heard the warning, but he didn't take it seriously. His report card, issued before the final two games of the season, showed two Ds. He still didn't believe that his dad would halt his basketball play. That night, after his dad got home and reviewed his grades, Skip was off the team. Skip was made to call the coach and explain why he wouldn't be able to play. The embarrassment was almost as painful as the disappointment. When the phone call ended, Tommy turned to Skip.

"Skip, I want you to know how disappointed I am in you. And for you. I wanted as much as you did for you to finish the season. Watching you play is a joy to me that you probably can't understand at your age. But your class work and your grades are the most important aspect of school. We haven't asked you to do something you can't do. We've asked only that you work and spend time with your studies. And you haven't done that. Now you pay the price."

It was the first time that Skip had approached a starring role; he couldn't understand how his father could deny him that. But it was denied.

The following year Skip tried out for the eighth grade football team. He was faster than his classmates, but smaller. He didn't make the team. His dad, however, helped him try out for the community league and he quickly learned the fundamentals and became a dependable running back.

He sat on the bench in eighth-grade basketball for most of the season and failed to make a letter in track that spring, yet he kept on trying.

His physique started to develop the summer before his ninth grade year. He landed a starting spot on the junior high school football team as an offensive end, but lost it before the season started to a transfer student. Still, he kept at the practice and the workouts at home, regaining his position and remaining in the starting lineup.

He failed to letter in basketball again and his football season the next fall was cut short by a broken ankle in the first game.

But he began to find himself athletically. He ran indoor track through the winter and was confident that he could make the spring varsity track team. He set his sights on his first varsity letter.

He remembered the excitement when he came home from school the afternoon that the members of the varsity team had been named. He ran up the steps, two at a time, and into his room, shutting his door to the rest of the family downstairs. He sat on the bed for a moment, more out of breath from pure elation than from the race to get home. When he caught his breath, he stripped off his clothes, leaving them in a heap on the floor, and walked to the mirror wearing the red-and-white varsity track uniform.

He adjusted the red shorts and tucked the white shirt deeper into the pants. He turned sideways, bent into the runner's starting-line stance, smiled at his reflection, combed his sandy hair.

For the first time in a long, long while, standing in front of the mirror, Skip Wilkins felt good. He'd made the team. A sophomore on the varsity track team.

The frustration and sense of failure from seasons past were gone. There was no room now in his thoughts for the broken ankle that had cut short the football season. No room for the fruitless hours he had spent on the basketball court, only to watch the game from the bench.

He knew that he was going to be a track star.

He flopped back on the bed, stared at the ceiling and thought about the past three weeks — the paralyzing nervousness he felt the first day of spring practice; the shyness and uncertainty of being around junior and senior lettermen whose names were known throughout the school; the puzzlement when he discovered that some of the best athletes cheated during the long practice runs, sprinting ahead of the pack and then hiding in the bushes to rest until the slower runners caught up; and, finally, the tinges of pride as he began to receive an occasional word of encouragement from a teammate or from Harvey Sergeant, the coach.

He thought back to the trial 440 that had won him the uniform. The day was rainy and only a few students and parents had shown up for the trials. No matter that the crowd was small. It seemed to him that the track's infield and stands were packed and that everyone was watching him, expecting him to stumble, to fall on his face.

He remembered the raw panic that set in as the starter raised the gun. And clearly, as though he were now running the race, he recalled the calm that overtook him as soon as he came out of the starting blocks. The practice — the lonely miles around the school track, the afternoon runs through the neighborhood — took over. His body functioned as a runner, an athlete. Even the pain — the shortness of breath and the ache in his lungs — was pleasurable. He had won; he liked first place.

He wondered briefly after that race whether Dave Grochmal was really as good as everyone at school said. And if he was so good, why hadn't Dave beaten him?

He looked at the clock on the dresser, rolled over and pushed himself up and off the bed, and began to dress for supper. He looked in the mirror one more time before going downstairs.

Skip had run every practice as though it were a race. The first meet with rival Kellam High was all he could think about in class, on the track, at home in his room, during a lull at the dinner table. He kept telling himself that he would do well. Perhaps even win.

Finally, the day of the meet. He couldn't remember ever being so nervous as he pawed at the track, getting settled into the starting blocks.

The gun sounded. He was out of the blocks ahead of the pack and in the lead. He was running hard and running well, coming into the first curve.

Then he heard it — feet behind him. Dave Grochmal passed him, running smoothly and effortlessly on his outside. Then a Kellam runner. And another Kellam runner.

He tried to make his legs churn faster, he shouted to them, faster. Even before the third curve, his breath was coming hard, his arms and legs aching as he tried to pull up with the leaders. When he hit the back stretch, he knew he wouldn't catch anyone. But the disappointment didn't set in until he crossed the finish line. It was a huge wave sweeping over him. He was angry. Hot tears stung his eyes.

Dave Grochmal was beside him, an arm across his shoulder.

"Good try," he said, and moved on. Skip suddenly understood that what he had heard about Dave, the way Dave paced himself and timed his move, was true. Dave was good and that Skip Wilkins had a way to go.

The next day at practice Coach Sergeant moved Skip from the 440 to the 880. He had been watching him closely during the past weeks, and he explained that Skip might do better in a longer distance.

Skip didn't understand all of the reasons, but he saw the move as a new chance to prove himself. He began to do just that.

The 880 was, as Coach Sergeant had said, Skip's race. He could maintain the same speed and pace as the 440. And he could keep it up the entire distance. Steady, even running, right up to the finish. He ran the 880 in the second meet and placed third.

He was part of the varsity now and he set his mind on winning races and winning a letter.

A comfortable pattern developed. He was a member of the team. He ran the practice sprints all-out, winning them more often than not. It didn't matter that some of his teammates were loafing during practice, he still took pride in winning.

As the season progressed, Skip focused more and more on a varsity letter. He never shared his goal, not even with his dad, but he would think often in class and always during practice about the feeling he would have, if he lettered as a sophomore.

The letter became the single most important aim in his life.

In early May, before the last two meets of the season, Coach Sergeant met with each member of the team to explain who had already made a letter and who still had a chance to earn one.

The letters were based on points earned during the season; three for an individual first place, two for a second, and one for third place. The members of the relay teams had to divide the points the team earned.

Skip needed only two points to letter. If he placed at least third in each of the last two meets, he could do it.

Norfolk's Maury High meet was the tougher of the two. The team had two of the best 880 runners in the state. Skip came in third in that race, crossing the line just behind Maury's two best runners.

He was confident of a letter now. His attitude was positive, he had long since become a true member of the team, and he knew how to pace himself, how to train, and how to win.

The day before the city meet, Coach Sergeant passed out new warmups. They were red with white trim and the word ''Cavaliers'' printed across the back. Skip had finally gotten a pair of Adidas running shoes, red and white, made of kangaroo hide. He remembered his first pair of shoes that season. He had ordered them through the mail. He hadn't known at the time that the rest of the team bought their shoes through the coach. Skip had bought leather shoes and they had gotten wet in the first race. Wet and heavy because of the leather and the leather soles.

Now he had it all. Good shoes. New warmups. The shot at the letter.

The night of the city meet the stands and the infield were jammed with parents and students from all the Virginia Beach high schools.

Skip took some easy laps on the inside of the track as the time for the 880 got nearer.

He had never seen so many people. The guns going off for the sprints and the other runners in their school colors added to the excitement.

Then he was listening to Coach Sergeant:

"Skip, Don Rhodes pulled a muscle in the 440. I've got to pull you from the 880. I want you to run the second leg of the relay."

Skip was heartsick. He had run the relay several times during the season, but it wasn't his event. He thought about the letter and he started to ask the coach what the change would mean. But Sergeant was gone.

Skip had to know about the letter. He ran after the coach and caught up with him.

"What about a letter?" he blurted.

He remembered only that Sergeant had said, "If we win the relay, you'll letter."

He tried to grab hold of the enthusiasm that always came with the members of the relay team. But it didn't come. He kept thinking about the letter.

The gun sounded in the relay. Skip couldn't concentrate. His mind was off the relay and on the letter. Then on the relay, imagining that he would have a lead, then lose it.

His teammate was rounding the backstretch. He was in the lead. Skip reached for the baton, felt it in his hand, and closed around it.

He was in the lead, thanks to his teammate. The crowd on the infield was yelling in his ear. He couldn't make out the words. They were just sounds, but the noise added to his confusion.

He tried to think of the race, tried to pace himself.

He maintained the lead going into the third curve, the 330 mark.

Going into the last 100 yards, he had settled down and was talking to himself, telling himself to push his legs, to run faster.

Then he heard the feet behind him. And the slight breeze that he always felt when someone passed him.

He passed off the baton and pushed through the crowd to the back of the stands. He looked back to see his teammate losing more distance.

He felt humiliation and anger. He had lost the lead on his leg. The team hadn't won the relay. He had been pulled from the 880. His race. He could have won that one. Certainly placed. That would have been enough.

At 15, his whole world was suddenly shattering again. He pushed through the crowd to a spot behind the bleachers and cried. No one had to tell him that he hadn't lettered. He knew.

He had come so close to leaving disappointment and frustration behind. He wasn't sure at that moment, that he had the spirit to try anything else again.

8

The rhythmic hum of the ambulance's tires as they rolled toward Woodrow Wilson and the quiet inside the ambulance kept Skip in a state of pleasant drowsiness. He slowly turned the collection of athletic memories in his mind, as hands might carefully turn a globe to view a different part of the world.

His failure to win a letter hadn't been the end of his young world. The summer sun had quickly bronzed him and burned away the disappointment of the track season. He spent his vacation running, working with weights, surfing and water skiing.

When he returned in the fall of 1965 for his junior year and another try at football, he was named the No. 2 left halfback. He became the starter in the second game; the first-string back had broken training rules and was off the team.

The third game of the season remained one of his happiest memories. Princess Anne had the ball for its second series of downs in the first quarter. Skip caught a flare pass in the left flat near the line of scrimmage. He dug his cleats into the ground, pushed off and sped upfield. He changed direction at nearly full speed to evade one defensive back, repelled the safety man with a stiff-arm, and outran two trailing defenders into the end zone. It was his first touchdown as a varsity player.

The score represented a breakthrough. He gained a confidence that had been lacking before. He became relaxed with his teammates, joining in the jokes and the locker-room kidding.

He ended the season as the team's leading rusher. He had become a threat on the sweeps and through the line. The newpapers referred to him as an "elusive, dazzling, open-field runner."

He received letters from three universities shortly after the season ended. Each said that he had the potential to play football in college and each expressed an interest in him, saying that he would be watched closely in his senior year.

He carried his new-found confidence into track season. He ran the 880 and the mile relay, lettering in indoor track in the winter and in spring track.

He was named the starting left halfback in his senior year. The team's offense was built around him and Charlie Shea, the fullback. More colleges began sending word through his coach, John Grady, that they were interested in him.

Even a sprained ankle, suffered in a pileup in the first game, didn't deter him. For the next three days, he watched every practice, leaning on a crutch. On Thursday, the day before the second game, he was able to put weight on the ankle. For the next 24 hours, he would one moment accept the fact that he wouldn't be able to play and, in the next moment, make up his mind to try it.

He showed up Friday evening in the locker room still not sure what to do. But the preparations for the game infected him. He wanted to play. He dressed for the game and ran several sets of sprints to convince the team doctor and the coach that the ankle was strong. It screamed with pain as he ran the sprints, but he was careful not to favor it.

He acted his way through the warmups and watched unhappily from the bench as Princess Anne bogged down on the first series of downs and punted.

On the second series, he was sent in with a trap play; he was to get the ball. As he ran toward the huddle, he kept reminding himself that the slightest indication of a limp would return him to the bench. He gave no evidence of the pain that he felt with each step.

As soon as he felt that ball slammed into his stomach, he drove for the hole that had been opened. He cut hard on the injured ankle toward the sideline as soon as he crossed the line of scrimmage. In the secondary, he dodged two defensive backs and had a clear field ahead of him.

For the remaining 45 yards, his gait alternated from a fluid run to a hobble as the pain drove itself up his leg and into his head. He crossed the goal line and let the ball drop to the ground. He limped back to the bench and the anguish on his face told Coach Grady and the doctor that he wouldn't play again that night.

Even with the sensitive ankle in the early games, Skip established himself as the premier running back for Princess Anne.

The team had won five consecutive games and Skip had scored six touchdowns and was the leading ground-gainer as Princess Anne readied for the final game of his senior year.

The seniors were keyed up in the locker room before the game with Cox High School. Skip was saddened at the prospect of not playing again with the teammates who had become such close friends during the past two seasons. He was, at the same time, priming himself to give this game everything that he could give. He didn't worry about the possibility of an injury. This was it. The last game of his high school career.

He scored twice in the first quarter, taking the ball in from the Cox 5-yard line for the first touchdown and outracing the secondary for a 35-yard score on the second touchdown.

Before the third quarter had ended, he had scored two more touchdowns, one on a 59-yard run that brought the Princess Anne fans to their feet, screaming for him to go all the way as he displayed his finest example of broken-field running. His last score came on a 10-yard pass to him. He had carried the ball nine times for 140 yards and ended his senior year with 60 points. Days later the statistics showed that he was the fifth highest scorer in the district. He was named to the all-district team.

The colleges started to woo him in earnest when the season ended. He received letters from 20 colleges and universities. All requested that he consider playing football for them.

College representatives began paying calls on Skip. Frequently he would be summoned out of class to meet with them in the athletic office. All had heard or read about him; some had scouted him. They all wanted him.

But they wanted something else, too, and that was a problem. Skip's grades were a solid C average, but he hadn't done well enough on the College Boards to meet the entrance requirements for many of the colleges. Several of the representatives counseled Skip to spend the next year in a prep school, where he could beef up his grades and continue to develop his athletic ability.

He discussed the situation with his parents and decided to enroll at Frederick Military Academy in nearby Portsmouth in the event that his approaching final try at the College Boards didn't improve his standing.

Shortly after football had ended, Skip added two events to his contributions to the indoor track team. They came about by accident. The team had been working out inside the school building during a cold and rainy afternoon. During a lull in the exercises, Skip approached and cleared a high hurdle that had been set up in the long hallway. Coach Grady had turned a corner of the hallway in time to see Skip clear the barrier with remarkable ease.

He asked Skip to try it again.

Skip walked back to his starting point, bent down in his starting stance, and again cleared the hurdle. He showed good form as well as speed.

Coach Grady set up a full flight of hurdles in the hall. Before the afternoon was over, Skip had become a high hurdler for Princess Anne in addition to a competitor in the pole vault, the high jump, long jump, 50-yard dash and relay.

He had a natural ability in the hurdles and began winning.

He entered the low hurdles for the first time in his life in the high school's district meet and he set records in both the high and low hurdles.

He co-captained the spring track team, leading it to first place in the city meet when he won the high and low hurdles.

His abilities on the football field and on the track caught the attention of Red Wilson, the newly appointed football coach at Elon College, a small four-year institution outside Burlington, North Carolina.

The coach offered him a scholarship which would continue each year if Skip could maintain a C average once he enrolled. Elon's requirements weren't as strict as other schools. Skip accepted the offer and withdrew from Frederick.

Princess Anne High School's awards ceremony, three days before graduation, crowned Skip's final year at school. In front of the whole student body, assembled in the football stadium, Skip was called forward to accept the trophy as the school's Athlete of the Year.

The determination and the work had paid off.

Graduation ceremonies were more important to his parents than to Skip. He was restless as he waited in line with his fellow seniors to march into the stadium on Friday night. Ahead was a two-day trip to North Carolina's Outer Banks and some of the best surfing on the East Coast.

As the line began to shuffle forward, and Skip, near the end of the alphabetically arranged seniors, began moving toward the seats set up in the center of the field, he became sad.

The feeling was sudden and totally unexpected. As he picked up his gait and began to cross the football field, the memories of the games, his runs, his pass receptions, and the friendships that had been born and had grown in the locker room filled his mind. For the first time, he realized that this night ended the happiest year of his life in athletics.

He thought about Pat. Pat Green, the captain of the cheerleaders, the good student, the girl whose name was written on his schoolbooks. He'd dated a lot of girls, but Pat had become *his girl* when he started his senior year. They had started dating after the first football game. Within months, they had become serious, perhaps too serious. Their feelings for each other had become too deep and too complex for either of them, at their age, to understand, and as time went on the relationship ended.

His first feeling of real love had left a taste of bittersweet. He doubted that he would ever forget her.

He tried to concentrate on the speaker's words, but his thoughts returned to football and track. He looked toward the bleachers, jammed with parents. His eyes sought out the cinder track, hardly visible because of the deep shadows caused by the floodlights. He pictured himself, left arm and right leg extended forward, parallel to the ground, clearing a high hurdle. The excitement about college turned into a pinprick of fright. He wondered whether he would be as good in college as he had been at Princess Anne.

"Alfred T. Wilkins Jr." The name boomed out of the loudspeakers and spread throughout the stadium. He had been watching his classmates, one by one, mount the platform and receive their diplomas. He hadn't heard the first name called. And now his name was being shouted, it seemed to him. Before the last sound of the 'r' in "Jr." had drifted into silence, he heard a collection of cheers, screams and yells from a section in the bleachers. He could recognize Linda's voice above the others. There they were once again, he thought, as he made his way toward the platform. His cheering section. The family that had urged him on, encouraged him when he was hurt and low and teased him back to humility when he had become cocky and smug. He mounted the steps and strode toward the principal who held the diploma in his outstretched hand.

As Skip walked toward the other end of the platform to return to his seat, he could hear Linda's voice, now clear above the polite clapping of the others in the bleachers, and the small, tight knot of Wilkinses who were clapping louder and harder and longer than anyone else.

The rest of graduation night became a series of pleasant detours on the way to the Outer Banks. The seniors had lingered after the ceremony, seeking out those who had been closest to them, embracing, shaking hands, offering good wishes.

Skip and Gary O'Brien, a neighborhood friend and surfing buddy, had stopped at Skip's home where the Wilkins family was waiting with cake and more good wishes. Patsy urged Skip and Gary to stay the night and drive to the Outer Banks the next morning.

"Mom," Skip said, with a new-found sense of independence, "you've helped me live my life for 17 years. I'm taking over."

Tommy smiled at both of them.

"He's right, Patsy. It's time. He's on his own now."

9

The Monday after graduation Skip was up early for work. During school he had worked part time as a stock clerk in a department store. Now he was starting his first day as a full-time sales clerk in the store's china department.

Gary O'Brien stopped by the store in midmorning to invite Skip to go water-skiing that afternoon.

"Why skiing?" Skip had asked. "The surf's got to be great this afternoon. The wind's been out of the west all night. The waves ought to be really shaped."

Gary left. When he returned, his persistence and the two attractive girls with him changed Skip's mind.

Skip had never skied on Lake Joyce, where one of the girls lived. The lake was extremely small, but he assumed that it opened into the Chesapeake Bay and that they would be skiing in the bay.

"Boy, what a boat," Skip said as he walked down to the dock. The boat had an 80-horsepower Mercury tilted out of the water on the stern. It was built for speed and pulling skiers. Skip was glad now that he had decided not to go surfing. The afternoon was going to be great.

His years on Currituck Sound had made him an excellent water skier. He felt more natural behind a speeding boat — pulling off to the sides and cutting the ski's edge into the water to throw up huge rooster tails — than on a surfboard.

The boat pulled away from the dock and followed the shoreline for a short distance to the right, heading toward a point. Skip thought the entrance to the bay would be around the point, but Gary stopped the boat and idled the motor.

"Skip, go ahead."

Debbie was getting her skis to throw over the side. Skip dropped the slalom ski into the water. Both were quickly ready to go. Skip nodded his head and motioned forward with his left hand.

Gary eased the throttle forward slowly until the tow ropes stretched out and became taut, then he gave the engine more throttle until Skip and Debbie, still in a crouch, broke the surface, found their balance, and stood upright.

The boat rapidly picked up speed and cleared the point. Skip could see that what lay ahead wasn't the entrance to the bay. It was just a large cove. He thought how small the lake was compared to the Sound where he normally skied.

The boat followed the shoreline of the cove, making a wide turn for a run in the other direction. Skip, on the outward side behind the boat, cut close to the shore, then out again.

As the boat made its run down the far shoreline, Skip began to use all of his ability. He pulled back on the two handles and leaned hard to his right, almost at a 45-degree angle to the surface. The shift of weight quickly sent him wide to the right of the stern, close to the shore. He shifted his weight now to the left and cut across the wake of the boat, coming out of the water on the single ski as he hit the wake. He was quickly across the stern and wide to the left of the boat, outside of Debbie, who was good, but indicated with a wide smile that she was impressed with Skip's ability.

He swung back, crossing the wake and swinging again wide to the right and close to shore. He was closing fast on a line of rocks just offshore and he began to shift his weight again in order to pull away from the shore and the rocks.

He felt a jolt.

His mind acknowledged that he was no longer holding the tow bar.

He was no longer in control on the ski.

He sensed incredible and uncontrolled speed.

The rest happened too fast and too suddenly for his mind to comprehend.

His ski had hit a rock just below the surface. The ski instantly had stopped slicing through the water. It was as if someone had jammed down hard on a brake. Skip was jerked out of the ski and up, into the air, before instinct or fear made him drop the tow bar. His 190 pounds, like a mass thrown from a sling, were hurtling through space, somersault fashion.

Then he slammed into the lake.

The impact left him with no sense of where he was or what he was doing. He thought some huge force had raised him up by his shoulders and smashed him, like a piece of glass, against concrete. The image of broken bones, smashed so small that they provided no more shape to his body, flashed across his mind. Then it was gone.

He opened his eyes. He was looking at water. Water that had been stirred by something. A stick, a hand. The water was churning and sandy. He could see bubbles rising. Above him, within easy reach, perhaps a foot, maybe more, he saw leaves.

Then he saw grassy stalks stretching upward, to either side of his head.

He was under water.

He couldn't move.

He couldn't feel anything.

Strangely, his mind registered no panic. He knew that he was hurt, perhaps seriously. His only thought was that he might never play football again.

Then he closed his eyes.

He felt a ring of air around his nose. But that was all he could feel. Then he heard the boat's motor, muffled by the water. The sound came closer and closer. He could make out voices, but he couldn't understand what the voices were saying. He had the sensation of bobbing like a log in the water, only his face above the surface. He couldn't focus his mind on anything around him.

He wondered if he were dying.

Or if he were already dead.

"Skip, you all right? What's wrong?"

"I'm hurt. I'm hurt real bad," he said.

"You're probably just stunned. You'll be all right. Just hold on. We'll get you up on shore. We're only a few feet away."

"No. Don't. Don't move me. I'm hurt bad." Skip could hear the two girls. They were becoming hysterical. They started to cry.

"Get a rescue squad," Skip said.

He heard movement in the water. Someone was leaving.

Skip turned his head slightly to the right to look at Gary, standing in the shallow water and leaning over him. Skip's right arm was draped over Gary's shoulder. Skip couldn't feel it. The arm was limp and awkward looking. He tried to remove it, to bring it back down by his side in the water. It stayed on Gary's shoulder. He tried again. This time he told himself to move his arm. It remained, limp and lifeless, across Gary's shoulder. The arm wasn't a part of him anymore.

Skip panicked. "I can't move. I'm going to die. I'll never play football again," he thought.

He began to sense pain. He had been numb all over, but now he felt as if someone were pushing hundreds of pins into his body. Then he felt a burning sensation. Both feelings started in his feet and he could feel them — the pins, the burning — moving up, until he felt the pain over every inch of his body.

Skip didn't try to talk. He tried only to keep his eyes open so that he could see Gary, who continued to lean over him. Gary was his only link with what was real and what was alive. Skip desperately wanted to hold onto that.

"Okay, fella. Take it easy. You're going to be all right." The voice was unfamiliar.

Skip looked up. A man in a white uniform was bending over him. Skip tried to smile at him; he was too weak now to try to talk.

The attendant and his partners eased a wire-mesh stretcher under Skip, using the buoyancy of the water to lift his limp body gently. They lifted the basket out of the water, careful to keep it level, and carried him to the ambulance. The attendant never left his side, holding Skip's head in a straight position on the 10-minute ride to the hospital.

The two men carried him into the emergency entrance of General Hospital of Virginia Beach and put him on an examining table.

Skip asked only once what was wrong. The answer was noncommittal.

A doctor began to work on Skip. He asked Skip to tell him when there was feeling. Skip waited for the doctor to start. Then he realized that the doctor was already moving along his body, probing with some kind of instrument. He wanted to feel something, to be able to tell the doctor that the probe hurt. He talked to himself, urging his mind to recognize pain, pressure, anything, just so he could tell the doctor.

"Yeah, I can feel it," Skip muttered. The doctor had worked his way from Skip's feet up to his chest. Skip had felt the instrument's prick near his breastbone. That was all that he had felt. He was relieved at sensing pain, but he was frightened that he had not felt the other jabs. The doctor was holding a large pin.

The doctor lifted Skip's right arm and began slowly to move the fingers back and forth. Skip looked at the arm. He felt nothing. It was as if it weren't attached to his body. The doctor moved around the table and repeated the exercise with Skip's left arm. Again, Skip felt nothing. He wanted to stand up. He knew everything would be all right if he could just stand up. He wanted to get up and everything would be all right if he could just go home.

The doctor moved away.

Skip was alone in the examining cubicle. He tried to remember what had happened, why he was in the hospital, where Gary and the girls were. The answers wouldn't come. He was on the verge of crying, but he was too scared. A high school graduate. On his way to college with a football scholarship. The thought of the scholarship and his football frightened him. He wanted someone to tell him that he was going to be all right. He stopped trying to be brave.

He couldn't remember how long he lay there alone. It seemed to him like forever. But the ugly nightmare was suddenly over. He heard a noise and opened his eyes.

His mom had arrived. She walked to his bedside and stood over him. She was telling him that he was going to be all right. That God would take care of him.

A tear came to his eye.

The memory of the accident jolted Skip back to his present surroundings, to the realization that he was on his back, paralyzed, riding in another ambulance to get help for his crippled body.

He squeezed his eyes shut and forced the details of the accident from his mind.

He wished alternately that the driver would hurry and reach their destination or that by some magic, something would happen to snatch him out of this bad dream and that he and his parents would suddenly find themselves at home and that everything would be normal.

But there wasn't any magic and the ambulance continued on the 200-mile trip to Fishersville and Woodrow Wilson Rehabilitation Center.

Part Two

10

The sunshine and the slight warm breeze felt good on my face as I waited for the stretcher to be pushed inside.

The building in front of me wasn't impressive; it was old and the brick was dulled.

But I was, in a way, excited to be at Woodrow Wilson. This was the place where I was going to walk again. I was anxious to get started. Whenever the word "rehabilitation" had been mentioned to me in Norfolk General, I had a vision of a stationary bicycle — the kind used for exercise, with no front wheel. I could see doctors and nurses helping me onto the seat, then working my feet and my legs so that the pedals began to turn. Then I would start learning how to make my legs work without help. I was prepared for it to take a while, but I knew that I would learn to walk again.

My excitement and expectations vanished as soon as I was rolled inside. The hallway was dimly lit and cool, almost cold. The walls were cinderblock, yellowed with age and badly scuffed. The odor of urine and the heavy scent of a disinfectant became stronger and stronger as we proceeded down the hall toward a room that would be my new home. I passed a dozen men, old and young, black and white. They had one thing in common: all were in wheelchairs. They looked at me as I was rolled by, but none of them spoke. There was no exchange of greetings, no acknowledgement of one another.

Even before I reached my room I was becoming confused, but the room and its sparse furniture pushed me past confusion and into fright. I wasn't going to be in a private room anymore. I wasn't going to have the individual attention that I had gotten in Norfolk. My bed was one of nine. They were olive green, but mostly they were chipped and scratched. There was no button to raise and lower the bed. A single hand crank was at the foot of each. There was no radio. No television. No button to call a nurse.

How was I expected to learn to walk again in such a place?

My mind was reeling at my surroundings when an orderly ushered my parents out of the room and stood over me as I lay in bed.

His voice was friendly.

"Well, let's see here, my man. We got to get you dressed so you can tour this place."

Dressed? I hadn't been dressed since the accident. And I'd refused to let Mom pack any of my good clothes. Somehow the clothes that I had taken so much pride in didn't seem right for the way I looked. Why would he want to dress me anyway, I wondered, just to sit in a wheelchair? I didn't ask or argue. I was too overwhelmed by this new place.

He peeled off my T-shirt and asked me if I wanted to put on underwear. He answered his question, not waiting for me. ''No, I doubt you do. Nobody in the infirmary does. It's a hassle. Especially when you have an accident.'' No underwear.

He pulled and pushed my limbs and rolled my body back and forth as he needed, bent and shoved each leg into a pair of pants and hiked the pants up to my waist. He explained everything he was doing to me as he worked. His words didn't register. I was sure he didn't know what he was doing. I was afraid that he was going to break my neck again. I'd never been treated that way.

After he had gotten my pants up and zipped, another attendant appeared. They turned me and partially lifted me into my four-poster brace. They quickly and casually tightened the brace and then lifted me out of bed and into a wheelchair. Just the two of them. In Norfolk, at least three and sometimes four attendants were needed to transfer me.

As soon as they had released me, I gasped for breath. The brace was too high and it forced my head back. The chair had a straight back, not a slanted one. The combination of the brace and the pressure of sitting upright for the first time began to choke off my breath.

I was struggling for air and fighting back tears. There was no way that I could survive, let alone get well, if this was going to be my treatment. I'll never do it, I thought. It's all over.

I didn't want to cry. I had been working to be calm. But the tears came. I lost my control and my ability to fight my feelings and I wept. My first time sitting up in this place and all I could do was weep.

The attendants, in gentle tones, tried to calm me. One of them quickly and easily readjusted the brace. The other kept patting my shoulder and telling me that everything was going to be all right.

Gradually I regained my breath and my composure. I was thankful that none of the family had seen me.

The tour of the center did little to lessen my apprehension. The rest of the main building and its furnishings were in the same state of disrepair as my room and my bed. There were three new buildings — a dormitory for vocational students, a dining hall and the recreation center with a swimming pool and television lounge. The family focused their conversation and excitement on the new things. We were all trying very hard to be encouraging and optimistic.

After Skip had been returned to his room, Tommy contacted the senior doctor on the center's staff. J. Treacy O'Hanlan was at home; he was usually at the center on Tuesdays and Fridays. The call to his home did not surprise him. O'Hanlan's job was to rebuild shattered lives and he needed all the help he could get, especially from parents. He would meet them at the center.

O'Hanlan already knew a lot about Mr. and Mrs. Wilkins. He knew that they were deeply caring parents, that they wanted to know everything about their son's condition and his needs, no matter how technical or complex, and that they had been supportive of the doctors and the staff in Norfolk. At the moment he found them more confused than apprehensive, but they were knowledgeable. It made O'Hanlan's first task easier.

"Mr. Wilkins, you obviously know a great deal about your son's condition. And about the prospects for his future. I wish more parents would ask the questions you apparently have asked. And learn the things that you and your wife have learned. It makes it easier on everyone. You, me, and especially your son.

"What Skip has injured is, indeed, the fourth, fifth and sixth vertebrae. They will never heal. He has lost the use of his legs. He has some use of his arms and only slight use of his hands. What we can do for him here is assist him in doing as much as he can to live his life. We'll help him learn to dress himself, to feed himself, to get around in a wheelchair. But that's about as much as we can do.

"He'll always be in a wheelchair. He'll always be on a bowel control program. He'll always be paralyzed.

"I can help to give him better tools than he has now to live a life; a productive life. But it's mostly up to you and to your son to provide the desire to use those tools. That's all we do here. We don't work miracles. At least not the kind that most people want.''

O'Hanlan paused, then went on.

''Do you want Skip to take up a trade? As you are aware, we also teach trades here once the patient has begun to learn to take care of his basic needs.''

Tommy answered. ''No. No, we're not interested in Skip's learning a trade. We want him to go to college.''

''Good. Then you should plan now for college next September. We will have done everything we can do for him well before then.

''Now, I know you're concerned, maybe even a little frightened, about leaving Skip here without your care. We don't look like much to most people. But we know what we're doing. And when we discharge Skip, he'll know pretty much who he is and what he can do. And with your help, he'll have a good life ahead of him. The best thing you can do is keep in touch with him. But don't visit too often. He needs to become independent. And call me anytime if you're worried or have questions. I'll keep you posted on his condition and on his progress.''

O'Hanlan had been part of that scene hundreds of times. He was always sincere and positive and, almost always, he was right about what he and his staff could do with the twisted human beings that came to Fishersville. As he drove back home from his office to take advantage of what was left of this beautiful afternoon, he sensed that he was dealing with a family who was going to match him victory for victory.

My introduction to the center had left me weak and exhausted. In the first hour, I had been dressed for the first time since the accident. I had been forced to sit absolutely upright for the first time since the accident. I had been bent, twisted, pushed and pulled as though there were nothing wrong with me.

I was back in bed, trying to collect my thoughts when the door opened. I looked up to see a fully clothed young man push his wheelchair into the room. We were alone and we looked awkwardly at each other for a moment.

''Hi, you're the new man, huh?'' he said, rolling closer to the side of my bed.

I couldn't take my eyes off him. He was a contradiction in this new environment. This place was supposed to help people get well. Yet here was a man, fully dressed and managing for himself and *still* in a wheelchair.

"Yeah, My name's Skip Wilkins. I'm from Virginia Beach. Why are you in that wheelchair?" The question came out before I meant to ask it.

He looked puzzled. "What do you mean? I broke my back."

"How long ago?"

"Five years."

I didn't understand. In a split second, I had asked another question, but it was a question that I really didn't want answered.

"Five years? And you're not out of that wheelchair yet? What's the matter with you?"

He looked at me as if I were crazy. That was his only response.

He rolled out and left me once again with my thoughts and the growing vision of my future.

Why hadn't this place helped him to walk again?

Was I going to be in a wheelchair the rest of my life?

I had thought often about the accident. I had acknowledged that my injury was serious. I had watched my once active and obviously muscular body deteriorate. But I had not really accepted the possibility of being permanently crippled.

Now, with that young man, it was different. It was believable. There was a person who had been injured, had been in rehabilitation and he was still in a wheelchair five years later. Five years or perhaps forever. Maybe it was just a matter of time until I had to face the fact that I would always be in a wheelchair, but at that moment I wished I could escape, could leave, could run away. But I couldn't. The place itself was forcing me to accept the idea of life as a cripple. If I could leave, get to a new and better place, I could get well.

My eyes began to fill with tears and the tears, for the second time that day, were ready to flood. But I wouldn't give in this time. I couldn't give up. I had to try. Maybe I would be different. Maybe I would learn to walk again.

The door opened and a large black man, dressed in a white uniform so small that the buttons strained, came in. He was pushing a young man in a chair. As they passed, both spoke.

"Hello there. I'm Junior," the black man said with a smile. "And this here, this is Tommy."

Tommy, a nice-looking, frail boy about my age, nodded shyly.

"I'm Skip. From Virginia Beach."

Before we exchanged any more information, Junior said he'd be back to me after he put Tommy in bed.

I smiled for the first time. With just a few words, Junior had introduced himself as a nice man.

He began the same procedure on Tommy that I had experienced when returned to bed. As I watched, I began to understand that Tommy's situation was like mine — he needed the same kind of help. Yet with him, the effort seemed to be part of a pattern; not awkward or embarrassing or frightening as it had been to me.

Watching brought some relief to me and the hope that maybe I, too, could relax and let the tugging and the pulling become part of a routine.

But as quickly as I tried to make myself comfortable with that idea, I had a terrifying thought. Someone was going to have to take care of me for the rest of my life. No, I told myself. No. As soon as that thought tried to return, I found something new in the room to study or to think about, forcing myself away from the negative idea.

Everytime I came close to getting a grip on myself, persuading myself that I had to fight back and I had to try, I met a new obstacle. A young girl who helped out at the center had fed me supper. It was obvious that she hadn't dealt with a newcomer before and I had no strength to help and no knowledge of what to do. She shoveled forkful after forkful of food at me, jamming the utensil so deeply into my throat that I gagged and the mashed potatoes oozed out of the sides of my mouth and down onto my chest. I became sick thinking of the sloppiness of the situation and the helplessness of my condition. I made a promise to myself right then that I would learn quickly to eat without help.

Shortly after supper, I became thirsty. A plastic jug filled with crushed ice and water was on my nightstand. I had not fed myself anything except grapes since the accident, but I decided to begin to learn. Besides, there was no one to help me.

It took a long time to lift the jar to my chest and to maneuver it close to my mouth.

Just as I thought that I was about to succeed in my first effort to help myself, the bottom of the jar slipped backward on my chest, pouring the contents over me and the bed.

I had an awful sensation. I could see the mound of ice on my stomach and the large wet areas on my T-shirt. But I couldn't feel the wetness or the cold. I wanted to move, to get up, to get out from under the mess even though I couldn't feel anything. Again, as my mind told my body to get up and nothing happened, I was reminded that I was paralyzed.

Junior came in and cut short any further self-pity.

"Damn, boy. Will you look at that? You ain't been here a whole day yet and you already causin' trouble." His tone let me know he wasn't upset. I wondered how he could have so much patience. I managed a weak smile and he smiled back.

"I'll be right back and we'll get it cleaned up. Better not be long 'fore you're drainin' that jug without spillin' a drop."

Those words, spoken by this big man whom I had known only a couple of hours, gave me something to grab. I had tried something on my own. I had failed, but he was telling me that eventually I'd succeed. And he was pulling for me to keep trying.

The next afternoon I met Chris Smith. I immediately had a warm feeling about him. I had heard about Chris before I got to the center. He was from Portsmouth, near Virginia Beach, and he, too, had a broken neck. He had suffered the injury while roughhousing after a touch football game.

He was spending some time with a family near the center and had come by to pick up some clothes.

He looked comfortable in his chair. He was nice looking and well groomed. Unlike some of the other patients I had seen, he had neatly cut, clean hair and was clean shaven. His clothes fit him well. His shoes were tied.

We chatted for a few minutes and then he rolled toward the door.

Before he went out, he turned back to me.

"Hey, Skip, take it easy for awhile. I'll see you later and we'll see if we can't get our beds put next to each other."

He smiled and lifted his hand as high as he could in a wave and was gone.

But he left something that was important to me. He left me the feeling that I had been accepted by someone else in this strange and still-frightening world and that he was going to be my friend. Now I had two friends — Chris and Junior. That thought didn't stay with me long after Chris left the room, but it represented a forward step simply because I allowed it at all. Hey, I thought, maybe this isn't going to be so bad after all.

Mom, Dad and my grandparents left me that afternoon. It was probably because I had just met Chris that I had a little confidence when they came to my bed to tell me goodbye. I was trying to view my stay at the center as a stay at football training camp, trying to make a team. I didn't know exactly what I was going to do at the center, but I was going to do whatever I was asked.

Dad told me that the doctor had asked them not to come back to visit for awhile. I started telling myself that I would be different — stronger and able to do some things — when they did return.

"Now you call Granny and Papa and your mom and me at least once a week," Dad said.

"We'll write and we'll be up as soon as possible."

"You can do it, Skip," he told me.

None of us that day knew what "it" would entail.

Mom leaned down and kissed my cheek. "I'll pray for you, Skippy. And remember, God is with you."

It was a good parting. When they left, I was excited about what lay ahead. I was beginning to understand that I had an uphill and pretty steep climb ahead of me, but I was building a determination to fight as hard and as long as I had to.

Tommy was the last of the family to get into the car. He slid his frame under the steering wheel and pulled the car door shut. He sat motionless for a moment, then reached forward and put the key into the ignition switch.

He fell back against the seat, trying to summon back strength that had suddenly left him. But all that came was a slow shake of his bowed head, and a single word, "Man . . ." It was spoken softly and it trailed off into silence.

Tears flooded his eyes and streamed down his cheeks as he sat behind the wheel, looking ahead at the red brick building that now housed his son and all his hopes for the future.

Patsy had been fighting her own battle against the rising tide of emotion. At the sight of her husband, normally so strong and determined and so seldom given to tears, she lost the fight and sobbed. Patsy's parents cried, too.

The four of them, who loved Skip so dearly and so deeply, shared a painful question that was articulated only by their tears: What will happen to him in this place?

I was taken to X-Ray on Monday so Dr. O'Hanlan could see for himself the damage to my neck. After he analyzed the films, he told me that my neck was in a stable condition and that I didn't need to wear the brace or even the collar.

I proudly relayed the news in my first phone call home.

The absence of the brace combined with the straight back of the wheelchair caused me to pass out the next time I was transferred to the chair. I hadn't had to learn, until then, how to breathe from my diaphragm. Without the brace to elevate my head and without the tilt to the back of the chair to keep the pressure off my diaphragm, I couldn't get air. My body adjusted quickly and when I regained consciousness, I was breathing without difficulty.

That same day I learned more about the importance of encouragement. I was sitting in a regular wheelchair with pegs on the rims. An attendant explained to me that my hands, despite their lifeless fingers, could pressure the pegs and turn the wheels. My first effort moved the chair from the bed to the door, about 20 feet. It veered sharply to the left because I had more strength on my right side.

Still, those few feet represented a big step forward.

The attendant patted me on the shoulder.

"That's great, Skip. That's just great. You'll be up and down these halls in no time." He said it in a way that made me want to succeed for him as well as myself.

On my first day, I was told I didn't need the brace and I was rolling my chair. I was elated at the progress.

I quickly got into a routine at Fishersville. I went to physical therapy each morning. At first I spent my time being strapped down and angled into various positions on a tilt board to rebuild my circulation. Then I began to develop and train and challenge the muscles that I still had to their full usefulness.

I had occupational therapy in the afternoon. I began to learn new and different ways of performing the simplest acts of living. In my second session, the therapist fixed a strap around the palm of my hand. There was a slit in the strap that helped me to hold a pen or pencil or fork. Before the end of my first week, I had managed to type a brief letter to my parents, slowly using the unsharpened end of a pencil to depress the typewriter keys.

As quickly as I learned to perform a basic function — eating with a spoon or fork, brushing my teeth, combing my hair — another challenge, always a little more difficult than the last one, was waiting for me — transferring from the chair to the bed, partially dressing myself. In each new task, I left behind as many of the medical aids and devices as I could.

The vision of the exercise bicycle that was going to help me walk again blurred and gradually disappeared. It was replaced by the reality of small weights that had to be lifted, of an object that had to be held.

Many of the everyday activities, like the morning and the afternoon therapy, became agreeable patterns in my life. There were other things, however, that were hard to accept.

None of us received much personal attention because of the vastness of the center and the small number of attendants and orderlies. I realized that there couldn't be much attention, but understanding it didn't diminish the desire for it.

Morning preparations for the nine of us in our one room were handled in mechanical fashion. There was only so much time to dress each patient and only so much time to help each patient groom himself. If I decided to stay in bed past the scheduled time to get up, I would lie in my bed, alone in the room for hours until someone found the time to help just me.

There was no privacy, not even for the most personal needs. Dressing and bowel training were accomplished in front of everyone in the room.

My first experience was degrading and repulsive. It never changed. Four or five of us lay naked on our bed pads while we were helped, by medication and attendants, to eliminate our waste. I clenched my teeth and squeezed my eyes shut as hard as I could. I was trying to shut out the reality of what was going on to me, with me and around me. Whenever the day came for the program, I had to talk to myself to get through it. Such things I came to accept as necessary, but I couldn't handle them without enormous mental effort.

11

As I struggled to overcome my fear and my confusion during my first days in the center, I began to think about God. I knew enough from my upbringing to believe that there was a God. I had been told over and over by my parents, beginning in the emergency room the day of the accident, that God would help me. I decided that I needed to establish a relationship with Him because I desperately needed help.

I made a commitment to Him, promising that I would pray to Him daily and would read His word if He would help me get better.

I was willing, I thought, to do anything to get well. So I tried to live up to my commitment. I got out the Bible that my parents had given me as a child and I started at the first page. I read and reread the story of the Creation and other passages, the same stories that I'd been told in Sunday school. They bored me. I kept trying, but something was lacking. Maybe my desire wasn't strong enough. Maybe I didn't understand how to go about what I had promised Him I would do. I began to feel that I was letting Him down. I decided that the best thing for me to do was not to bother Him at all, though I somehow always knew He was with me. I just didn't know how to reach out.

I wasn't able to draw strength from God, but I did find strength in some people. Chris became an important person in my life. He was more severely injured than I. He had no movement in his arms and wrists. I, at least, had some arm and shoulder movement and there was some strength in my wrists. He was a constant reminder that I could have been much worse off. He gave me something more important, however, than feeling thankful for my condition. He had learned to be positive about his future. He had learned to try and never give up. Because I knew that I had use of more of my body than he, I always tried harder than he.

As Chris and I became closer through the weeks, we discovered that we had something very special in common. He had developed a strong relationship, outside of the center, with one of the therapists. I had become attracted to Sally, who was in charge of my occupational therapy.

Even at the outset of the therapy sessions, her encouragement was important to me. I wanted to please her. I soon began to feel that she was interested in me as a person as well as in my development as a patient. She frequently spent more time working with me, staying closer to me than to the other patients. Her smiles of approval to me seemed warmer than those to the others. She often would give me a pat of encouragement or put her arm around my shoulders and hug me after I had accomplished some therapy task.

After a surprise party on my 18th birthday and after the others had left the therapy room, Sally gave me a present. Then she kissed me. It wasn't just a friendly birthday kiss. Sally was an attractive female and I began to realize, because of the way she apparently felt about me, that I still had emotions and I still wanted to be cared about and loved.

We began to spend time together away from the center. We enjoyed being with each other, we enjoyed the touch of one another and, as the relationship deepened, we kissed and embraced on our dates away from the center. I don't know that Sally and I were in love, but I know that we did have serious feelings, emotional and physical, about each other. Her internship at Woodrow Wilson ended shortly before Christmas and she left to work in another part of Virginia.

We knew that we would probably not see each other again, but our mutual feelings marked an important part of my physical rehabilitation: I began to believe in myself as a person. I began to believe that I could be attractive to other people again.

Granny and Papa always had been special to me and gave me and my sisters the little extras that Mom and Dad could not afford. Their visits to see me at Fishersville deepened my appreciation of them. Their hearts went out to those around me as much as to me. When they went to Rowe's Steak House for a suprise steak for me, they came back with steaks for others. It became a gentle joke among the patients: "I'm hungry. When are Granny and Papa coming to visit?" It had to be expensive, but they never stopped the practice. Their visits always meant some of Granny's homemade chicken and rolls — for the entire room, of course.

My ability to type a letter, punching one letter and then another with the pencil, gave me a special connection with Karen and Shirley. They wrote to me in the large scrawling hand of their age and I wrote back on the typewriter. It gave me the feeling of being a big brother away at college.

Tommy's small and secret diary on his son had less frequent entries now that Skip was separated from his family and telephoned only once or twice a week.

The entries since the day they had left Skip at the center and had come home to wait and hope pointed to progress:

> 8-27 No brace. Eating well. Working hard.
> 8-29 Typed two letters. FEEDING SELF. Gaining weight.
> 9-1 Pushing wheelchair some.
> 9-2 Visited. Looked good. Gained weight.
> 9-14 Went to circus. One person got him into car.

All of the entries were cryptic notes of good news — until September 21.

I suffered a setback on September 21.

Nearly four weeks after I arrived at the center, I had started on bladder training to end my need for a catheter, which drained into a plastic bag clipped to my right side. Once I had succeeded with the training, the catheter would be replaced by a snuggly fitting rubber sheath with a tube running to the leg bag. The catheter, because it was a foreign object inserted inside my penis, represented a constant potential for bacteria and urinary tract infections.

The training seemed simple when it was explained to me. The doctor would remove the catheter. I would be required to drink at least eight ounces of water each hour that I was awake. I was shown how to hit myself in the bladder area; the slight blow would trigger the bladder, forcing it to empty completely and properly.

When I actually practiced what I had been told, it didn't work. I forced more liquids. Within a short time, my bladder started to swell, pushing itself against my stomach. My stomach became distended. My repeated blows to my bladder area failed to make me void. Within hours, I had fire-red splotches over my body. I became chilled, then I broke out in sweat from the internal sickness. I ran a fever.

I had to stop and the catheter had to be reinserted. I tried again the next day, and the next, without success. The constant efforts and constant failures to train my bladder were slowly causing uremic poisoning.

The poisoning finally made itself obvious. I developed a high fever that didn't break, even with the catheter reinserted. I was taken from the center to the hospital at Staunton. I was packed in an ice bath until the fever dropped, then I underwent minor surgery to crush the kidney stones that had developed in my bladder.

When I returned to the center, I tried the bladder training program again. Again it failed. For the next several weeks, I was in and out of hospitals: first at Staunton, then at the University of Virginia Hospital in Charlottesville. I became familiar with the routine of treatment: first the ice baths, then the minor surgery to crush the stones, then back to Woodrow Wilson.

My efforts at bladder training were no longer continuous. The sickness had slowed, then interrupted, and finally halted the rest of my therapy.

I was caught in a horrible medical dilemma. I needed to train my bladder to remove the catheter and its potential for disease, but each effort at training brought on uremic poisoning.

The feeling of helplessness and frustration came back. I had been fighting so hard to get better, to take care of myself. The sickness brought the end of moving ahead. I wondered whether I had anything left to give. Each time I asked the question, I looked at the others who had so much less than I did and I thought of my family and how much it would mean to them for me to get better. Somehow, I was able to dig deeper inside and try again.

During this period, people at home — outside of the family — started to become important to me.

I temporarily halted my bladder training and went home for the first time at Thanksgiving. Mom and Dad had worked to make everything just right. Dad had built a small ramp at the front door for the wheelchair. Linda had moved all of her belongings upstairs to my old room, Karen and Shirley had moved into Linda's room, and Mom and Dad had taken the two girls' room. I was given my parents' first-floor bedroom, the largest in the house. Dad had hung pictures of my football and track performances on the wall.

My new room had been completely furnished by Leonard Strelitz, who had helped Dad find out about Woodrow Wilson. He was a highly successful businessman and owned, among other things, a large furniture outlet. The Strelitz' affection for the Wilkins family went back to Papa's generation, when Papa and Granny had been helped in the early years of their marriage by Mr. Strelitz' father. A bond of friendship and respect had developed between the two families and I was the latest beneficiary with an entire bedroom suite.

Karen and Shirley were my constant companions. I wasn't able to pull myself up in bed or do much else without help. They stayed with me, waiting on me and watching television with me. Their attention made me feel that they had missed me and needed me as much as I missed and needed them.

Linda was in and out of the house with her own social life, but she would always stop by before going out or come in to see me after her dates and tell me where she'd been and whom she'd seen.

But my homecoming was not the happy occasion we had anticipated. I felt awkward. At Fishersville I was like the others. At home the people were different. They could walk. When I went home I realized that Mom and Dad would probably have to do all the things for me that attendants were now doing at the center. They had already done so much. Yet there was so much ahead for them to do, no matter how much better I became.

I was invited to a party for the football team at Thanksgiving. Martha Chevalier, the girl who I had been dating before the accident, came over to talk to me almost as soon as I arrived. She looked great, more cute than pretty, and she had a nice figure. I had written her several times from Fishersville. She had always responded quickly, telling me how much she wanted to see me when I came home. Her letters were friendly and mostly about what she was doing and questions about me. There was never a lot of news about other people. I didn't know how she would react to me in a wheelchair even though we had been dating just before the accident.

She came to the house to visit after the party. Because of my experience with Sally, I continued to hope that one day I would have a relationship with someone. Someone like Sally or Martha. We didn't talk that night about seeing each other in the future, but I felt that she wanted to be with me. Our letters became longer and more frequent when I went back to Fishersville.

Wayne Whitley was at the party, too. He had played tackle on the football team and had been one of my classmates. We hadn't been too close when I was at Princess Anne, but he came by the house several times during Thanksgiving and we kidded and talked about football. He had been ineligible to play his senior year and I had worked to get him elected president of the Varsity Club. He didn't know that and he came to visit, I suspect, because he was something of a loner and he knew I'd become something of a loner, too, because of what had happened.

When I returned home for Christmas, Martha, Wayne and Wayne's brother Mike, who had helped Linda so much when I was in Norfolk General, were the first people to visit. Martha and I dated during Christmas in the only way that I could. She visited in the evenings and had dinner with the family. We would watch television and talk in the privacy of my room.

Wayne borrowed football films of the games in my senior year and brought them over. As I watched myself on the screen, healthy, strong and running, the question of playing again kept coming back to me. I kept answering the question, ''no,'' but I still hoped, without reason, that my athletic career wasn't over.

Except for the visits from Martha, Wayne and Mike, Christmas was a sad time. Our family tried hard to make the holiday as much like past Christmases as they could. But we tried too hard. The strain, especially on Mom, was beginning to surface. After we opened our presents on Christmas morning, an awkwardness filled the house. All of us knew that, because of the concern about too much activity for me, we would not be riding to Papa's for a traditional Christmas Day breakfast and more presents. I couldn't take my mind off the thought that my presence had brought an end to one of our most cherished times as a family. I tried to be happy and light-hearted, but I kept thinking about the burden I had become. Christmas of 1967 was the worst Christmas that we had ever had.

I returned to Fishersville to resume my therapy. The center had halted my bladder training after the repeated failures and the repeated fevers and trips to area hospitals. I remained on the catheter.

Dad called in the spring with a possible solution to the problem. He had located a Norfolk urologist, Eugene Poutasse, who had practiced in rehabilitation centers and had successfully performed the required surgery many times. I had known for some time that Dad had been trying to find a doctor but I never thought about it. I had begun to dislike hospitals because of what they meant to me. And I had almost come to accept the fact that I would need to have a catheter, with its potential for problems, for the rest of my life.

I left Woodrow Wilson Rehabilitation Center on June 1, 1968, nine months and 13 days after the ambulance from Norfolk General had stopped outside the dull brick building in Fishersville, Virginia, that had become my world.

I didn't know whether or not I would return as a patient. The decision would be based on the success of the scheduled bladder operation and how well I could get along at home.

Robert Smith, one of the older patients who had been in and out of the center for 13 years because of a paralyzing accident, didn't make my departure very easy. He wanted to give me some advice that he thought would help me when I left.

"Skip," he said, "be prepared to make new friends when you get home. Your old friends' lives have gone on since you came here and they won't be there to help you pick up your life."

I argued with him.

"You don't know how many friends I have. They'll be there to help."

A sadness came to his face and he gently shook his head.

"I hope so, Skip. I sure hope so."

Dr. O'Hanlan saw me shortly before I left. He had the same kind of advice.

"Skip, you have a lot of potential. But you've got to remember one thing, if you don't come back here: be prepared to change for the world. Because the world won't change for you. It doesn't owe you anything."

The advice from Robert Smith and Dr. O'Hanlan tempered my

happiness at being discharged. There were reasons to be happy. Physically, I was stronger. I had gained back 25 pounds and I weighed 145.

I was able partially to dress myself.

I could feed myself.

I was able to push my chair, to get around on level surfaces.

Mentally, I was able to acknowledge my present limitations. I continued to hope for a way to improve, but I recognized that I was bound,
at least for a while longer, to a wheelchair.

I didn't want to accept the counsel that I had been given, but I had
learned that Dr. O'Hanlan knew a lot about people in my condition. I
filed away his words, hoping that I wouldn't need to be reminded of
them.

The operation on the bladder was called a TUR — transurethral
resection. It required trimming some of the muscle out of the neck of the
bladder so that the muscle would respond to internal or external pressure, such as the blows that I had been instructed to deliver to myself.

I woke in my room after surgery and looked down at the urine bag
clamped to the side of the bed.

The bag was nearly filled with blood-tinted liquid. Dr. Poutasse
came in and assured me that everything had gone well.

Days later the catheter that had been inserted following the surgery
was removed and I again was put on a training program. Dad sat beside
me in the hospital room as I drank cup after cup of water.

The symptoms that I had come to recognize so well began to return.
My bladder started to distend once more. I began to splotch. I could feel
myself getting warm, then hot. I broke into patches of sweat. I hit my
bladder area over and over. Nothing happened. I was becoming
panicky.

Nurses put me in a tub of warm water. Still nothing happened.
Finally they put me back in bed.

"I'm afraid we'll have to put the catheter back in," one of them
said.

When they left, I told Dad that I wanted to try something.

"Dad, I don't want that catheter back in. Come over here and press
down real hard on my bladder. I saw it done at the center.

He was hesitant at first.

"Where? What do you mean, Skip?"

I explained as well as I could.

"I've got to somehow trigger my bladder off. You push down real hard on my stomach." I showed him where.

"How hard?"

"Hard. Right here."

He pushed.

I felt a sensation inside my body.

"Push again. Harder."

He put one knee on the bed beside me and pressed again.

Fluid, a mixture of blood and urine, trickled out. We both saw it.

"Push again."

He did. This time the urge to void gave way to another trickle. Then a stream.

I was voiding. I mean *really* voiding.

The two of us must have looked ridiculous; a grown man, clothed from tie to shoes, straddling a young man, lying unclothed in bed, and pushing on his stomach. And then the voiding.

We didn't feel ridiculous, though. The two of us knew what had happened. The operation had worked; I would be able, with practice, to trigger the emptying of my bladder and to leave behind the catheter, one of the morbid reminders of my condition. I would be fitted with an external device which had no perils of infection or discomfort.

One of the nurses returned to the room. Before she could take in the sight and understand what had happened, I told her that she wouldn't need to bring the catheter.

12

I was home and there were no problems staring me in the face. The nine months at Fishersville had helped me develop my muscles and my ability to get along with little assistance. The stay at the center also had built my determination to tackle yet unforeseen obstacles. The operation in Norfolk had eliminated the need for a catheter. My emotional outlook was healthy.

During my first weeks at Fishersville, I had built up a fear of coming home. I worried about the things that Mom and Dad would have to do for me the rest of my life. Only days after I came home from the TUR operation, that fear had completely gone. It had been erased by the way Mom and Dad had handled my needs. During the weekends near the end of my stay at the center, I stayed with them in a motel outside Fishersville. Dad had been the one to help dress me and undress me. Mom had watched. When I had gone home for my first visit at Thanksgiving, Mom had begun to assist. Now that I was home for good, Mom assumed the full responsibility, freeing Dad during the week to concentrate on his job. The changing of roles had been so gradual and so smooth that I had hardly noticed. Mom and I were comfortable working together each morning and each evening.

Wayne Whitley's visits during June represented some of the best medicine that I received. He treated me as though nothing had happened to me and he was always encouraging me to go out with him to visit and be together with other people.

One afternoon in late June, I overheard Mom talking on the telephone. She was telling someone that she couldn't leave the house. Only Shirley and Karen were home and there was no way that I could be put into the car to ride with her.

When she hung up, I rolled into the room.

"Mom, come on. I can go with you."

"Skippy," she said, "you know I can't lift you. Even with the girls' help. You can't get into the car."

"I watched a lot of people at Fishersville getting in and out of cars without being lifted. We'll put my transfer board on the car seat and I'll just slide from the chair into the car. Then we can leave the chair here. Come on, let's try it."

She thought about it for a moment, then smiled.

"Okay, if you think we can."

I told Mom and Shirley and Karen what to do, remembering the transfers I'd seen at the center. The girls slid one end of the long narrow piece of wood under my chair seat and rested the other end on the car seat. I was awkward and slow; I had never tried to transfer without the help of someone, like Dad, who could lift my weight. Slowly, putting weight on my knuckles and arms, I was able to shift my body along the board while the girls held the board. Finally I rested, somewhat awkwardly on the car seat. Mom lifted my legs into the car and Shirley and Karen put the wheelchair in the house.

As the Volkswagen pulled away from the house, I left behind one more barrier. That day we won my freedom to travel, a freedom that had become precious to me only when it was no longer mine.

Linda, now 17, became my chauffeur and all three sisters became my constant companions and my closest friends during the summer. We drove to the beach nearly every day. The heat was a problem for me because my body no longer adjusted to it. I could perspire only in response to sickness, not external heat. I passed out several times on our trips to the beach before we learned to carry water and ice with us. We always went to the beach near a place that offered me air conditioning if I became too hot in the sun. Shirley and Karen would push me along the boardwalk or sit with me inside a restaurant or snack bar when the temperature forced me out of the sun.

August came and brought with it another effort by Dad to find a way to help me. He had been working to have me evaluated at the highly acclaimed Albert Einstein Institute in New York City. Leonard Strelitz, who had been so helpful, knew about the institute and had worked with Dad to have my condition evaluated. Dad was determined to try anything available to help me.

Dad told me that the doctors at Albert Einstein Institute had made a preliminary study of my records. They thought there might be a bone chip pressuring my spine that could be removed. If that were true, I might regain the use of some of my muscles.

I went back to Fishersville for a final checkout and Mom and Dad drove me to New York. I was to undergo 21 days of tests.

I had mixed emotions as I prepared for the trip. So much had happened to me in the past year. So many ups, so many downs. Every-time there appeared a hope of a normal life, I came out of the situation with new evidence that my life in a wheelchair would be permanent.

But I kept on hoping. Maybe someone at some place would be able to do something. Maybe at Albert Einstein. There were endless questions churning around in my mind. But the one thought that managed to creep in more and more often was the thought that maybe, just maybe, something could be done. And if not, I hadn't really lost anything. I knew that we had to go and find out.

Einstein was different from any place that I had stayed. The doctors talked with a hint of optimism. They spoke openly of a possible bone chip in the fourth vertebra. If they could remove it, I might get additional return in my limbs. They talked of the possibility of braces for my legs.

I had a large, semi-private room. My schedule was typed out and given to me. It included every test that I could think of: X-rays, muscle evaluation, occupational therapy evaluation, bowel and bladder evaluation, a myelogram, wheelchair evaluation and brace evaluation. They wasted no time. On my second day there, I started 21 days of consecutive, thorough testing of every part of my body.

From the beginning, the tests challenged me. A nurse, a therapist or a doctor was always with me, encouraging me to hang on, to be a little more patient, to undergo just one more test that day. I fought the weariness and put forth all the strength I could find for the evaluations. I wanted to show them how much I could do.

My final evaluation at Einstein was with leg braces. It was a new experience.

A therapist and an attendant strapped my legs and lower back into a complicated brace of metal and pads.

As they worked with the brace, I looked up at the parallel bars. I knew I would be carried to them in the next few minutes.

This, I thought, is what I had first thought rehabilitation was all about. Someone would stand me on my feet. Once up, my legs would take over. I would begin to shuffle my feet. I knew I would be slow and clumsy at first. Then I would take small steps. Finally, I would begin to walk. That had been my impression of rehabilitation.

That thinking had been changed by my stay at Fishersville. No matter. I had in front of me my first opportunity to stand since the accident.

I listened to the therapist as she told me what was going to happen and what she wanted me to do.

My heart beat with excitement as I thought about standing up.

The attendant locked his arms around my chest and lifted me to the bars. The therapist kneeled down and locked the braces at my knees. I looked at myself in the large wall mirrors in front. I was standing. But the image I saw in the mirrors sickened me. One of my feet turned in. My shoulders were pushed up above my neck as I pushed against the bars. The braces were the worst part. They were big and clumsy looking, hiding my legs. I looked like a cripple.

The attendant backed away. So did the therapist. I was now on my own.

"All right, Skip. Lock your arms at the elbows. And lift with your shoulder muscles. You want to try to raise your feet off the floor."

I tried to follow her instructions, but I couldn't. I pushed against the bars as hard as I could for a few seconds. What little strength I had in my arms and shoulders were gone. I had just barely lifted my feet. The effort drained me. I nearly passed out. I was carried back to the chair.

I sat exhausted, staring into the wall mirrors and thinking about what had happened. My arms and shoulders ached. I was completely drained. My body throbbed out the message of how difficult the brief test had been.

I didn't have the strength to hold myself between the two bars. There would be no more attempts. The test was over and I wasn't going to walk or even stand. The guarded hope that I had brought to Albert Einstein flowed out of me along with my physical strength as I sat in the chair. I had looked a cripple in front of the mirrors. I began to accept the fact that I was crippled.

I was still weak from the efforts at the bars and I was beginning to suffer ill effects from an earlier myelogram as I sat with Mom and Dad.

The doctor was summing up the long days of testing.

"We have been unable to find a bone chip. There isn't anything else we can do here for Skip.

''But the results are encouraging. His attitude is excellent. He can physically do more than we would expect for a person with his type of injury. It is possible, with surgery, that he can gain additional use of his hands.''

The doctor continued to paraphrase for us the test results that were on the desk in front of him. I heard only words and partial sentences, but I knew what he was saying:

''Continue life as he is now . . . handicapped in a normal world.''

His message was clear and he spoke it with courteous and sensitive finality.

''Go home. Prepare for the future. Start school immediately.''

Tommy and Patsy had talked a lot about college for Skip. They had agreed that he should go as soon as possible, depending on the results from Einstein. Those results were in now and it was Tommy's responsibility to tell Skip.

He had waited almost a full day after returning from New York. Skip had remained ill from the myelogram on the drive back to Virginia Beach.

The findings of the myelogram were conclusive. The results had been conveyed just before Skip was discharged. There was no bone chip that was creating pressure. No bone chip to be removed. In short, there was no hope for improvement in the spine.

Tommy had been encouraged by one finding at Einstein. There was a possibility, the doctors said, that a tendon transplant might give Skip more use of his hands and fingers. Tests had detected residual life in each hand.

Tommy filed away this information in his mind and his notebook. The hands could wait. College was immediate. Tommy expected Skip to balk at the idea of college so soon. But he knew that his son was going to be in a classroom that fall. A college education was imperative to help insure a future for Skip.

''Skip,'' Tommy began that night after supper, ''you know your Mom and I have been checking on college for you. I think we ought to do exactly what the doctors suggested. We ought to start right away.''

Skip wanted to say something, but Tommy continued.

"I've checked into colleges around here and there is one that I think will meet our needs. It's a small one over in Chesapeake. Chesapeake Junior College. All of the classrooms are on one floor. The dean of students, his name is Thomas Russ, said that he would be happy to have you as a student. He wants to meet with us as soon as he can. Classes start in 11 days. I have an appointment for us tomorrow."

Now he stopped. He could see that Skip wanted to speak.

"Dad, that sounds great. But maybe we ought to wait a little while. Until I'm stronger. The second semester would be better, don't you think? It wouldn't be as hot and I'll be even better adjusted."

Tommy disliked the role he sometimes had to play in his son's life. He was the heavy. The unpopular messenger of the unpopular things that had to be done. When he and Patsy discussed the future and when the two of them decided on a course, no matter what kind of advice and reaction he got from others — and it was sometimes unpleasant — he was going to see it through.

"Skip," he said, "we've got college *now*. We're here together and we're all going to help. We've got to do it."

The girls chimed in, as if on cue from their father.

"I'll be able to take you in the mornings, Skip, before I go to school," Linda said.

Shirley and Karen promised to help their brother with his assignments, doing whatever writing and typing he would need.

There was no further discussion. Skip's apprehensions remained but, as he had nearly always done, he was going to follow his father's advice.

Tommy looked at his family, gathered around the dinner table. That was one of the payoffs. The family had come together and closed ranks again, this time around Skip and college, just as they had closed ranks when the blow had been struck against them on the bottom of the lake. It was that payoff that sometimes kept Tommy going, that reminded him that sacrifice and hard decisions were worth it.

13

Football was on my mind as Mom, Dad and I drove the five miles to Chesapeake Junior College for pre-registration. Football had been the reason, before the accident, that college had been important to me. Athletics was out of the question now; college held the unpleasant promise of only books and classes; Chesapeake didn't even have a football team.

I began to acknowledge how important this step was to my future. I wondered whether or not I could succeed in the classroom. Studies had been unimportant to me in high school. I lived for football and track.

I was shocked at the campus as we pulled to a stop. It was small. It looked more like a house on a big lot. One building, one floor.

Thomas Russ changed my disappointment. He was cordial to us and very proud of his college. I found myself caught up in being a college student. When he had finished going down the list of possible degrees, I kept thinking about one that he had mentioned early in his conversation: counseling. I had seen so many people helping others in the past year. That was what I thought I could do and do well.

I was enthusiastic when I explained that I thought a career in counseling, particularly involving young people, was the proper one. I had seen and had received so many people's efforts to deal with others' emotions during the nine months at Fishersville. When I finished explaining my choice, Mom, Dad and Dean Russ were in agreement with me.

That night, alone, I thought more carefully about what had happened during the day. Events had moved faster than I could keep up with them. My earlier enthusiasm about a counseling career now gave way to the immediate future: getting around to classes; no friends; no study habits. That night before I fell asleep, I kept telling myself that I couldn't let anyone down, least of all myself.

I was scared as Mom came to a stop in the college parking lot on my first day of classes. The lot was crowded, people were everywhere and the campus now looked large and foreboding. I was nervous as I transferred to the wheelchair. I was conscious that several students would glance my way, then look away when they saw me looking at them. It was an awkward beginning.

Small ramps had been placed at each doorway to the buildings. I was the only wheelchair student at the college. They had been built for me, by direction of Dean Russ.

Mom's goodbye was brief.

"I'll be here to pick you up at noon. And, Skippy, I'll pray for you." With that blessing, I was on my own as a college student.

I felt self-conscious in class. Other students took down pages of notes as the instructor lectured. I couldn't write. I was relieved when the class was dismissed early, but even more relieved when the instructor came to me with an assuring smile. He discussed my special needs, including the use of someone's notes and taking exams on an electric typewriter. He made my first day a little easier.

A student met me as I neared the door to leave the building at the end of classes.

"Can I give you a hand?" he asked.

"I sure would appreciate it. The ramps are a little steep for me."

He smiled and helped me out.

I made my way down the sidewalk that surrounded the school. The students now spoke easily and naturally to me. Their casual friendliness helped more than they knew.

Mom drove me home. I was tired, mentally and physically; but I felt good about myself and my first day at college. I had made it through on my own.

About this time, Dad and I took a trip that stirred some deep memories.

We went back to the football stadium at Princess Anne. I was returning to see a ball game.

When we pulled into the parking lot, I suddenly was back in school as a student. A Friday night in the fall. I could hear the cleats scraping along the parking lot as I saw myself walk with the team from the dressing room to the edge of the field. It was an eerie feeling and an emotional one.

I hardly heard what Dad was saying to me as he pushed me toward the end zone. People stopped us along the way. They spoke to me, told me how glad they were to see me, and told me how much they had enjoyed watching me play.

It was a haunting feeling. I sat near the end zone and looked onto the empty field bathed in floodlights, where I had made a name as a player and where the team would soon appear. Some of my runs and touchdowns on that field came back to me. A sadness that I hadn't experienced for a long time returned.

I wondered what might have happened if there had been no accident.

Someone stopped to speak and interrupted my thoughts. As they left us, the familiar drum roll began. I instinctively looked to the goalposts. I knew the team would be lining up there to run onto the field for pregame calisthenics. They were there. I knew what was going through their minds. The nervousness that came before each game and that didn't disappear until the first play was called, the first contact made.

The drum roll gave way to the sound of the full band playing. The team sprinted between the goalposts and onto the field. Some of the players looked my way. There were a couple of waves and a couple of "thumbs up" signs in my direction.

Even if the lights had been better, I wouldn't have known who the players were. My eyes were full of tears.

While my return to the football field had a deep emotional impact, my return to my church had little impact at all.

Except for my one brief try at praying and reading God's word in the early days at Fishersville, I had been without any spiritual influence or interest.

Now the influence was present, but the interest remained absent. I attended church with the family. I continued to believe in God; He had been a major part of my upbringing. But I didn't have a personal relationship with Him. I knew that He was out there somewhere, perhaps looking down on me. But that's about as much thought as I gave it.

Church became more a hindrance than a help. I recoiled with a sense of dishonesty whenever people at church would come up to me and claim that my courage and my determination were fine examples of one of God's people. I became annoyed and even angry at the number of people who came to me to share stories about friends and relatives who suffered similar accidents and who recovered through prayer and God's healing. I didn't know what God had in store for me, but I couldn't see how He was going to heal me. All I knew was what I had heard over and over: prepare for a future life, Skip, with what you have now.

I wasn't comfortable with the example that friends in church believed I was setting.

I wasn't comfortable with the idea that God might have a plan to heal me.

I tried, whenever I could and with whatever excuses I could find, to avoid a religious life altogether. But I tried just as hard not to let Mom and Dad know my feelings. That, I felt, would have been the biggest blow to them since the accident. Especially to Mom.

Mom, more than anyone else in the family, had enough burdens now that I was home. She was the primary caretaker for all of my needs.

The strains that the accident and my rehabilitation and my present condition had brought into the house showed from time to time. Tempers would flare, sometimes over the smallest things. One morning I lashed out at Mom simply because the cuff to my pants leg had become twisted, showing the top of my sock. She hadn't straightened it and I couldn't. But we were quick to forgive and we wouldn't allow anyone to brood over problems. As a family, we fought the tension and we tried to drive it out of the house as soon as it surfaced.

I was beginning to make friends at school. I went to keg parties and drank my first beers. I'd never wanted alcohol before. It had never been in our home. It wasn't even discussed. But almost everybody in college drank and I tried it out of self-consciousness and a need to be accepted. The thought of what was waiting for me at home after my first drink, if either Mom or Dad detected beer on my breath, made me stop for chewing gum before the night was over. It wasn't long before I stopped the drinking.

I also began to have a social life at home. Dad had bought a pool table for me. It was one of the things I could do from the wheelchair. The garage was his special place, the place where he went to be alone and to tinker. I knew the place meant a lot to him. After we picked out the pool table, he took up his tools and his projects from the garage and set up the table. The garage soon became a special place for me and for a growing number of friends. It was the first activity that I could participate in with other people. Before friends started dropping by, Shirley and Karen learned to play and would spend hours with me so that I didn't have to play alone.

There was a girl in my life, too. Throughout 1968, the year that I returned home, Martha had become the most important person in my life. Despite the fact that we had dated when I had received so much attention as an athlete, she accepted me now as I was. During the weeks with Sally at Fishersville, I had begun to hope that I could be loved by someone outside the family. Martha was turning that hope into a reality.

I worried about not being able to take her out easily, but she assured me constantly that those things didn't matter; that she was happy just being with me, whether it was helping me with schoolwork or being out with others. I was still trying to accept fully my disability and I wasn't persuaded always by what she said. I often picked arguments with her about trivial things and expressed doubt about her feelings for me just to see what she would say. I tested her affection continually, even in the face of all she did for me and all she meant to me.

There were times when physical feelings, as well as emotional ones, seemed very natural. On those occasions I allowed myself to think about Martha being a part of my life forever.

In January of 1969 a member of the Cosmopolitan Club of Norfolk paid us a visit. His name was R.E. Dorer and he had heard about me through his wife, who knew Mom. He explained that his organization undertook an annual project to provide help to an average family which suddenly found that it needed assistance. The club was interested in finding out whether I had some need that it could help fill. Dad told him about the practical need to enlarge my room to provide study space.

Mr. Dorer then spent some time talking alone with me. He wanted to know about my plans for the future and he also asked me to outline my ideas for a complete room of my own.

He left, saying he would be back in touch.

Several weeks later he returned. The Cosmopolitan Club wanted to build an addition to the house. Not only would I have ample space to study, but I was to have a roll-in shower. No longer would Mom and Dad have to carry me from my chair, through the narrow hallway and into the tub. Construction would begin as soon as we could provide the plans.

In the summer of 1969, our place in Carolina lured me back. It had represented fun and shared moments of happiness with the family until the accident.

My first trip back, the summer of 1968, had been painful. I sat looking over the waters where I had skied, run the boat and fished. That day, all I could think about was a future without those things that I enjoyed so much. On a later visit with Martha that summer, Uncle Ackie and Dad rigged a lawn chair in the boat for me and I went cruising with them on the sound. It whetted my appetite for the water.

Now Bill Milleson, a friend in college, helped change those year-old feelings of frustration about not being able to go boating. He had lost interest in a small haul-seine boat that he was building and he had offered to finish it for my possible use.

I was excited. I approached Dad about the idea and he took to it instantly.

Bill and Dad got some help on the project. Linda's boyfriend, Jamie Spencer, and Mike Preziotti, a friend of Bill's, put in flooring and rigged a steering system. A 10-horsepower motor was the finishing touch to the boat. The four of them mounted a crane on the side of the dock with an old boat winch to lower me aboard, seated in the wheelchair, and lift me out.

As I was lowered into the completed boat on a beautiful summer day, I realized how fortunate I was to have a family and friends who worked so hard for a gift that meant so much to me.

The boat opened another freedom for me — I could once again control myself on the Sound. It brought back to all of us a sense of happiness about Carolina.

The return to Carolina also toppled a psychological barrier for the family. Dad had lost interest in boating after the accident. He was especially reluctant to take the girls water skiing. It reminded him of the accident and he also felt that if I saw the girls on skis, I always would be reminded of what had happened to my life.

Linda and I bought a slalom ski for Karen and Shirley to use. We gave it to Dad one night after dinner and told him it was for the girls. He didn't say anything, but he looked at me for a long time. I knew that he was asking me if I could handle the image of one of my sisters on the thing that had crippled me. I nodded to him. The single ski reopened a world that had been shut to all of us and the summer became one of the happiest that I ever had. I felt that, in some small way, I had given something to the family that had given so much to me.

The Cosmopolitan Club completed the work on my room addition in November 1969 and I gained another measure of independence. I had my own entrance, plenty of desk space for typewriter and books and plenty of room for the wheelchair. Most happily, I had a shower room large enough to accommodate me in the chair and to end forever the need for someone to lift and carry me to the tub.

Martha had returned to Longwood College for her second year and we developed different sets of friends and activities and interests. Our letters became less and less frequent. I began to push her out of my life. On the few occasions that we saw each other in the fall, our relationship was definitely different. It was altered because I wasn't confident enough to believe that we could make it together and I didn't want to cause her unhappiness in the future. Our closeness was going to end.

We saw each other for the last time as a couple during the Christmas holidays. It was difficult for both of us. She meant so much to me, yet I believed that I was doing the right thing — for her sake and for mine. I missed her the moment she left our house on the last day that we saw each other. I hoped that one day in the future I would be able to accept love, like Martha's, that was given without concern for my condition. But I knew that this wasn't the time.

The sadness over Martha was countered by a joyful Christmas morning. After the family had opened presents at home, we drove to Granny's and Papa's. The visit was both a family reunion and a Christmas celebration. Auntie and Uncle Ackie were present for my first traditional Christmas breakfast since the accident. Conversation and laughter filled the house from the moment we arrived until we left that afternoon.

The trip to Granny's was only 12 miles, but as I thought back on our somber Christmas of 1967, I realized that all of us had traveled closer to becoming a whole family once again.

14

A nightmare greeted me on my return to college for the second semester. Another quadriplegic had enrolled in the fall. I had read in the newspaper about his death during the holidays. I learned the details on my first day back. He had taken his own life.

He and I had been similar in some ways. We had about the same degree of physical limitations. Both of us were tackling college head on, maneuvering around or rolling right over the small problems that cropped up.

There were some differences between us. His parents had provided for him in a way that my parents couldn't. He had a specially equipped car. He had his own home that had been customized for his handicaps. He had a small swimming pool in the yard. I must have had the one thing that he needed. I had the desire to keep on living, even if it was in a wheelchair. For many days after learning of his death, I thought back thankfully to the discipline, to the emotional strengthening that I had received at the hands of Dr. O'Hanlan at Fishersville. I thought about my parents who had given me their bedroom, about Dad who had given up his private place in the garage. My whole family had given themselves to me, helping me to find courage when I lost it and to keep my determination close at hand.

I thought how tragic it must have been for my schoolmate. To have had so much and yet not enough. I knew that his parents, who had tried so hard, must have felt pain and frustration. My heart went out especially to his sister, no older than my own sister Karen. She had found her brother and the shotgun and the yardstick that he had used to reach down from his wheelchair to trip the trigger to end his life.

I vowed, no matter what happened in my future, that I would never put my family through such an ordeal. Out of this almost unspeakable tragedy, I found one more reason to keep on.

15

Daphne Via walked back to her bedroom still thinking about the phone call. As a student at Princess Anne, she had known about Skip Wilkins. She had never been introduced to him. But the whole student body knew his name. He was one of the most popular people in school. The good-looking football star. Kind, never cocky. He was two years older than she.

She had heard about his accident after graduation. She remembered the benefit dance for him that had been held at school.

None of that, however, explained why she had agreed to go on a date with him, given her present frame of mind.

She was outgoing and attractive. She'd dated a lot at Princess Anne, but it was never anything serious. She simply enjoyed the popularity that her looks and her personality had brought her.

Lately, however, she was subdued and was not interested in going out. She had just broken up with a steady boyfriend. She focused as much of her attention as she could to her classes at nursing school. She was too lonely and depressed to think about men right now.

Why Skip Wilkins then, she wondered again? Could it be pity? No, it couldn't be. He was good-looking and he certainly seemed to be having fun when she saw him across a crowded room at a party some months earlier. Besides, she didn't know enough about him to feel anything for him.

She remembered being caught off guard at that party by Linda, Skip's sister, whom she had known at Princess Anne. Linda had asked if she would accept a date with Skip if he asked her for one. She had glanced in his direction. He was sitting in the wheelchair, surrounded by several couples.

"I guess . . ." She had caught herself quickly. "Sure. Yes. Of course, I'd go out." She hadn't been comfortable with her answer. It had been an awkward moment. But she couldn't bring herself to say, "No."

Now, out of the blue, five months after seeing him at the party, he had called to ask for a date and she had said yes to him.

She started to become apprehensive about the date. She'd never been out with anyone in a wheelchair. She tried, without success, to imagine what she and Skip Wilkins would do on a date — especially at a

Friday night school dance.

"Well. Daphne," she said to herself as she brushed her hair, "you'll just have to see. You accepted the date and you certainly can't back out of it."

Friday was four days away.

Don Pollard was driving his van. He, Rob McClintoch and I were headed for the dance. Their dates had fallen through at the last minute and I was embarrassed about taking Daphne without any other girls. But there was no turning back.

We stopped for beer and then for Daphne.

Don went to the door. As I watched him go up the walkway, I felt insecure that I couldn't call for her and meet her parents. And this was the first date. I realized how nervous I was.

As I was worrying about all of the things that I wanted to do and couldn't, Daphne appeared at the door of the van.

"Hi, Daphne, I'm sorry that I couldn't . . . ."

"Don't worry about it. I understand," she said. She smiled and climbed in and we quickly fell into a conversation about mutual friends, days at Princess Anne, and what we now were doing. She was instantly easy to be with and a lot of fun. We enjoyed the dance, talking and joking, almost nonstop. The four of us decided to ride to the Beach after the dance. Don and Rob went off to one of our favorite spots to drink beer and Daphne and I continued our conversation alone in the van.

She was sitting on the back seat of the van and I asked if she would like for me to join her. When she said yes, I began to transfer from the chair to the seat, something I hadn't done before in a van. She amazed me. She held the chair and offered assistance, easily, without fumbling and without awkwardness.

All I could think about as we continued to talk was how much I wanted to kiss her. She was so pretty and so comfortable to be with. I knew, after only a few hours, that I liked her very much and that I wanted to see her again.

My desire to kiss her was slowed by questions that I hadn't asked myself since the accident, despite other dates.

I wondered how she'd react, whether I would make some awkward move and be embarrassed. For some reason, it was very important that Daphne Via be impressed with me.

But the desire finally won out. I had to try.

I leaned toward her and she leaned to meet me. It was a gentle kiss. My arms were around her and I held her for just a moment before it ended.

Daphne eased the front door shut behind her and leaned back against it for a moment. "He's nice. And good-looking," she thought. "I really had a good time. And all we did was talk."

She thought about the kiss and worried about it. "I shouldn't have let him kiss me. Not on the first date. I wonder if he'll ask me out again."

His condition hadn't bothered her. He had handled it well, never mentioning his limitations after his effort to apologize for not being able to come to the door for her. He seemed confident and out-going, but kind and genuinely interested in her and what she was doing. She liked the feeling she had with him and the warmth that had come over her when they had kissed.

She was positive that she didn't feel any pity for him. Maybe it was a reaction to the hurt that she had suffered from her recent breakup. No, that wasn't it. It was something about Skip Wilkins. She wasn't sure exactly what it was, but she knew that she wanted very much to see him again.

Shortly after my date with Daphne, I went to a Princess Anne High basketball game. Karen was a cheerleader and I was beginning to follow her career at home games just the way she had followed my football games and track meets.

During halftime, a man came over and introduced himself.

"Skip. I'm Larry Via."

I was taken by surprise. When he realized that I was confused, he said in a bold, clipped way, "I'm Daphne's dad. You dated my daughter last weekend. Remember?''

Before I could answer, he went on.

''She had some nice things to say about you. I've read about you, too. If there's anything I can ever do for you, you just let me know, you hear? And come back to see Daphne soon. And meet the rest of her family.''

I was overwhelmed. On the next date, Daphne brought her mom, Helen, and her dad out to the van to meet me formally. They reminded me of my first meeting with Daphne; they, too, made me feel comfortable in spite of the fact that they had to come to the van to meet me.

Several weeks later, I was invited to a Sunday supper at the Vias. Daphne picked me up in her family's stationwagon. Mr. Via came to the door to lift the chair up the steps to the front porch.

''Skip, we're going to have to build a ramp for you,'' he said matter-of-factly.

When I rode with Daphne to her house for my next visit, there was a ramp going up to the front porch.

''Daph, that's really nice of your dad.'' That was all I could say. I wanted to say much more. The ramp meant to me that I was accepted, wheelchair and all, by the Vias.

My life became a busy combination of attending class and dating Daphne.

College broadened into an active social life. New friends visited, shot pool, and stayed at the house in the evenings to talk, watch television or listen to records. Mom and Dad allowed cards to be played in the house and occasionally we played poker until late into the night. Friends would often be invited to stay for dinner. Life was similar to my high school days. In the early days of my return home, I remembered what Robert Smith and Dr. O'Hanlan had told me when I left Fishersville. They had been right. Many of my old friends had gone on with their lives while I was away. I had to accept myself and had to form new friendships with people who would take me as I was.

Daphne and I saw each other several times a week. We double-dated almost all of the time because of the transportation difficulties. Don Pollard and another classmate, Nancy Schmidt, became close friends and we spent much of our time with them.

Mary and Paul Bradley became very important to Daphne and me. I had met Paul at our place in Carolina when I was six. His parents lived in Norfolk and had a summer place near ours. Paul was older than I, but during the summer he would take me on hunting and fishing trips and let me run with him as he worked out. As I matured, he and his wife became my close friends. Paul and Mary settled in Norfolk after their marriage. I wanted very much for the Bradleys to like Daphne. I was becoming serious about her.

Paul and Mary and their four children lived near Norfolk's DePaul School of Nursing where Daphne was enrolled. Paul would pick Daphne up after her classes, I would get a ride to the Bradley's and the four of us would fix dinner together and enjoy the evening.

Now that I was dating steadily, money became a problem. Since the accident, Mom and Dad always made sure that I had spending money. My grandparents frequently helped. My need had increased and I was embarrassed about having to ask each time I dated.

Mom became my sounding board to solve the problem. She knew, but never said, that my feelings for Daphne were becoming stronger. As it always happened, Mom passed my concerns to Dad. That night he helped me solve the problem.

"Skip, I'm going to give you $15.00 a month from now on. But I know that you'll have special things come up for you and Daphne. And there're going to be times when something unexpected happens. I want you to come to me when that happens and I'll try to help you out."

Papa and Granny also began to give me a monthly amount. The allotments weren't large, but Daphne and I found enjoyment in planning together what we could do with the money.

Daphne and I weren't uncomfortable about my condition. After our first date, we talked frequently about my limitations and my needs as we planned to go to parties or to be with friends.

Daphne had learned about some of my physical problems and my requirements in her nursing classes; others came up in our conversations; and still others became a part of what linked us together as a couple rather than separating us.

I had become accustomed to the sheath and the leg bag, but I was sensitive about them around Daphne.

Often when we were out with friends, I would excuse myself to go outside to empty the bag, always asking one of my male friends to accompany me. I was unable to bend down far enough or pull my leg up high enough to unclamp the drainage tube at the bottom of the bag. Daphne insisted that she could help me, that there was no need for me to be sensitive about it.

One evening, when I needed to excuse myself from the table where we were talking, she followed the two of us outside.

"Skip, I can help you with that," she said.

I turned to Don. "Okay, Don. We'll be in in a minute."

Daphne easily unclamped the tube to drain the bag, straightened my pant leg, and pushed me back inside as if she had performed the task hundreds of times.

I didn't say anything about the incident then, but I thought how fortunate I was to have someone who was so willing to share all of my life — including the problems that had come with my disability as well as the fun and joy I was beginning to experience.

The weekends during May of 1970 at Carolina brought me three gifts.

Daphne had accompanied Mom and the girls to Carolina to clean the trailer for the summer months. I had told her of the pleasures I had found there for so many years. I wanted her to find enjoyment there. She returned with an understanding of why Carolina was special to me and with her own appreciation of the land and the waters of Currituck Sound.

During the first weekends at Carolina, Daphne and Linda became very close friends. The two of them stayed in Granny's and Papa's trailer and they would stay up late, talking and baring their feelings. I loved the two of them very deeply and in different ways and I felt a real joy as I watched the two of them growing to care about each other more and more.

My third gift satisfied a desire I had experienced the previous summer each time I saw a bass boat.

Bass fishing had always meant a freedom, a serenity and a competition that bound men together. I could not remember a summer before the accident that I had not had a bass rod in my hand. Now, with no grip in my hands, I couldn't hold, let alone handle a bass rod.

Watson Stuart, a summertime friend at Carolina, and Paul Bradley helped me take up fishing again. It wasn't bass that we were after; it was white perch.

Even with the limited ability in my hands, I could cradle the pole loosely in both palms. Because the cane pole had no flexibility, as a bass rod did, and no reel, I was able to lean back and jerk the pole to hook perch. Watson or Paul would set the proper length of line and set the bobber at the proper height for the depth of water we happened to be fishing in.

Sometimes we would drop anchor; other times just drift in the boat.

When we decided on a spot, those of us in the boat — sometimes two, sometimes three of us — would beat the water rapidly with the poles to imitate the sound of schools of minnows rushing through the water. White perch are one of the few fish that are attracted and not frightened by sound. Within minutes, one of us would feel the first fish hit the hook.

From then on, if the school of perch had followed the lead fish, we'd hook and jerk the catch into the boat. We sometimes caught as many as 50 fish in 10 minutes. Often Daphne went with me. She became adept at taking fish off my hook so I could return my line quickly to the water. Mom taught her how to clean the fish.

I'd had a full day on the water on June 26, a Friday. Daphne had arrived at Carolina that afternoon and we were happy because she had finished her nurses' classes for the semester. She had a job in the emergency room at General Hospital of Virginia Beach. Most of the summer still stretched ahead of us.

The family had settled for the night. As was our custom, Daphne and I were resting on my bed in the living room of the trailer. I was dressed for bed and under the bedcovers. She was propped up next to me, lounging on top of the covers. The moon was full and it beamed through the large window that overlooked Currituck Sound. There was a sparkling pathway of light across the water.

"Daph," I said. The words came out softly, the way a person sometimes talks to himself. "Could you see yourself spending the rest of your life with me?"

There was a brief silence, then she slowly propped herself on one elbow and looked down at me.

"Are you asking me to marry you?"

"If you think that we can make it, I'd like to give it a go."

She started crying and we held each other very close and very tight.

"I don't know when I can get you a ring," I said. "I don't even know when we can get married. You have school to finish and so do I. I don't even know if I can get a job when I finish school.

"You know we'll have a different kind of physical love than other couples, and I have no idea about children. But I know that I love you and that you're the person I'd like to live the rest of my life with."

Never in my life had I felt so good about anything. Daphne Via, beautiful and bright, full of life and love, was excited about becoming my wife.

I broke the quiet that fell over us.

"Daphne, can't you just see it?" I said in the same soft and thoughtful voice, which now was contrived.

"We'll be married here at Carolina. Maybe on the pier. We can have the guys holding pole canes. That's it. We'll go under an arch of pole canes."

We laughed at the image.

"I don't care," she said, "when or where or how. I just know that I want to marry you, Skip Wilkins."

16

The pleasured days of summer slowly gave way to fall.

I was eager for classes to begin. I was in my final year at Chesapeake Junior College and I felt confident that I would be ready to transfer to a four-year college and get a full degree.

I rarely thought about my confinement to a wheelchair now. There were other things to occupy my mind. I had friends, good grades and a growing sense of my own worth. I had been elected vice president of the student body earlier in the year. It hadn't been a tough campaign; we had no competition. But the president, Bill Milleson and I did generate some excitement and some enthusiasm for the school.

Our biggest and most successful campaign ploy took place the night before election day. The college had no flag pole on campus. Bill had salvaged a 25-foot pole used to hold fish nets in the Chesapeake Bay. We gathered together some of our "campaign staff" — we had enlisted the aid of all of our friends at school, assuring a victory even if we had had competition — and spent the midnight hours installing the pole in front of the main entrance. I didn't give a second thought to the fact that I was wheeling around in the dark, giving directions and providing encouragement to a dozen classmates; I did acknowledge to myself that I was thoroughly enjoying the escapade.

Once the pole was in place, we hoisted an American flag. The next morning the flag was waving in a steady breeze as students arrived. Low on the pole we had attached a painted sign, " Contributed by the Milleson and Wilkins Campaign." The flag, to the delight of students and many of the faculty, flew daily the rest of the school year.

I concentrated on my studies and my life. Daphne and I spent all of our free time together. We continued to be frequent guests in the Bradley household and at our favorite spots at the beach. Whenever I went out socially, I went with Daphne.

If it is possible, I was feeling contentment in the face of permanently limited physical life.

But my contentment and the serenity that had settled over life in our home was suddenly shattered on Sunday evening, January 17, 1971.

I was lying alone in my room. For no apparent reason, I felt very tired and weak. The cause of my fatigue became apparent about 6 p.m. when Mom started to drain my leg bag. There was no mistaking what I saw. I had blood particles in my urine, an abnormal and frightening development.

I soon became nauseated. I knew that whatever was wrong was serious; my body was sending me that message with the vomiting, the splotches of sweat, the chills and the aching.

Dad measured the amount of fluid that I had been able to pass during the evening: three pints. Three pints out of five quarts of water that I had had. I wasn't passing as much fluid as I should be. He was worried and so was I. I called Daphne to tell her that I was leaving for Norfolk General, that she shouldn't worry and that I didn't think it was anything serious. But I really needed for her to tell me to be calm and not to worry.

Dr. Poutasse wasn't available, but his intern was. I was in excruciating pain by the time I reached the emergency room. I vomited again. My bladder continued to distend and I could get no relief. I simply couldn't void. I was almost glad when the doctor said that he was going to insert a catheter to enable me to void and to relieve the pressure building up in my bladder. I was in so much pain that the psychological fear of the catheter didn't come.

My bladder emptied. I felt as though I had just finished the hardest-hitting football game of my life. My upper chest, my shoulders, my neck, my head and my arms ached.

The doctor said I could return home. Both Dad and I were worried. We didn't know what had caused the problem and we didn't know whether it would return. The doctor tried to assure us that he didn't believe that it was serious.

As I lay awake that night, I knew something was definitely wrong. I could sense it. As if to endorse my fear, my body heaved and contracted and I vomited again. Only this time nothing came out. I hadn't eaten since lunch. I exhausted myself wondering what the next day would bring and I fell asleep.

I awoke without the chills and fever that I had experienced the night before. I was able to void. I tried to eat, but couldn't. It was difficult to force liquids down. The problem, whatever it was, was still there, I thought to myself.

By 10 a.m. Monday the chills returned. I tried to force more liquids, hoping it would ease the problem. My temperature began to climb — by 1 p.m. I was on my way to the hospital again.

The examination in the emergency room was long and extensive. Intravenous pyelograms (IVPs) were taken and I was put on intravenous liquids and given antibiotics.

By early Monday evening my temperature had stabilized at 101 degrees. After several more hours of observation and no reduction in the fever, I was admitted to Intensive Care. It was 10 p.m. I was exhausted, frightened and sick. My surroundings added to my fear. I was back in the place where it had all begun less than four years earlier.

I tried to eat the next morning, but I couldn't keep anything down. My heartbeat was rapid. I had never experienced any problems with my heart and I was scared. With each beat, I thought my heart would explode and burst through my chest. It was as though someone were inside pounding against my chest with a sledge. Soon, a throbbing headache accompanied the pounding of my heart. The harder my heart beat, the more frightened I became and the stronger the poundings became.

A specialist in internal medicine was called. Each minute added confusion. I underwent more X-rays, then an EKG. I began vomiting again although there was nothing in my stomach to empty. I was catheterized again and the pounding and the pressure in my head and heart lessened for a short while. I returned to a private room.

Tuesday night a private nurse came to stay with me. I was too weak to ask why she was there.

The next three days and nights seemed endless. I was barely aware of the visits by Mom, Dad and Daphne. I still had blood in my urine and my heart and head had not stopped the constant and fearful pounding. The doctors finally isolated the potential problem. They performed a cystoscopy and found infection in my bladder. They changed my medications and ordered stronger sedatives to provide some relief from the constant pains in my head and upper body.

Slowly I began to respond. Dr. Poutasse was now treating me. I felt secure in his care because he had helped me so much before.

Two more days passed and the problems diminished. On Sunday, January 24, one week after the problem had begun, Dr. Poutasse released me and instructed Dad to bring me back to the hospital at the first sign of any problem.

I was home for three days. On Thursday, the chills returned with the fever, the nausea, and the aching. By 7 p.m. that night I was back in the emergency room, this time rushed there by the rescue squad. As I lay in the back of the vehicle with its red lights rotating outside and the siren bleating as we approached an intersection, I thought back to my ambulance ride in June of 1967. I had felt then that I was going to die. Once again, I felt that I was close to death.

My temperature registered 105 degrees when I was admitted to Intensive Care. I was given antibiotics and put on an ice mattress. For the next three days, medicine and constant supervision of my vital signs were my whole life.

Once again the fever began to drop. Finally it returned to normal. On February 2, after five more days in the hospital, I was well enough to be sent home. I stayed at home for two days, then tried to return to school. I couldn't make it. I was too weak. Professors sent assignments home and I tried doing the work in bed. Daphne visited as often as she could, but she had her own schoolwork. When she couldn't visit, she called and sent cards. Her visits and her messages bolstered me and I managed to hang onto some will to get better.

Late in the night of February 7, the chills and the fever came back. The next morning I was back in Intensive Care.

I had first become sick on January 17. It was now February 8. I had been taken to the hospital four times in 23 days. I was in Intensive Care for the third time in three weeks. As I lay in bed that night, weak and afraid, I cried out to God.

"Why?" I asked Him. "Why? Why now? When I've accepted my accident. Why are these things happening to me? Why more problems?"

I had never called out to Him before, but I was scared and I was desperate. I couldn't understand why I was being punished again. What had I done to deserve this sickness and this pain? Only God, as I understood Him, could do this. And surely, I thought, He must have a reason.

Three days and nights passed with no improvement. I was growing steadily weaker. There had been other times that I had been depressed:

in the room in the C Wing, looking at the leg dangling awkwardly from the bed beside me; at the center, on my first day; when I couldn't make my bladder perform. I had somehow managed to work my way back to a positive attitude from all of these. But now I had nothing left to fight with. I was so tired. I felt defeated, mentally and physically. The fever continued. I had constant and severe chest pains. My heart and my head increased their pounding each time my bladder tried to drain, even with the use of the catheter.

Mom was sitting next to me by the bed that night. I think she knew that I was ready to give up.

"Mom," I said, "I don't know if we're going to make it this time."

When my words came out, we both felt fear. It was the first time that I had ever admitted the possibility of death.

She reached for my hand.

"Skippy, you *are* going to make it. Of course you are. We're with you. Your dad. And the girls. And me. We've come so far. All of us. And you have Daphne to live for. She cares so much for you."

Mom was giving me the last bit of strength that she had saved for herself. Usually it was Dad who exhorted and encouraged, not allowing me to give up. Now here was Mom, talking so quietly, and so surely, giving me reason and resolve to keep fighting, when I was at my lowest point.

Tears came and so did some last, small measure of strength.

It was enough.

Patsy felt so helpless. She wanted more than anything else to give her son that night the strength to keep on fighting and keep on living. She would have traded her life away in an instant to insure his. But she knew that God didn't barter, that He always had a purpose in His plans. Earlier that night, she had tried with all the faith and all the love that she, as a Christian and a mother, possessed to tell her son that he was going to live. But she knew that only God could help him.

Patsy glanced at Daphne, sitting next to her and staring ahead as the car headed toward DePaul Hospital and Daphne's room. She was glad that Daphne had been able to forsake her schoolwork and to visit Skip for a few minutes. He had managed a weak smile when Daphne entered his room.

This young woman, Patsy thought, means so much to my son. She knew that the two of them were serious about a life together. She had known that even before Skip announced to the family that he had asked Daphne to marry and that Daphne had said ''yes.''

Patsy was worried for Daphne almost as much as she was worried for her son. She felt that she had an obligation to Daphne, even if she risked hurting Skip.

She eased the car to a stop in front of the nurses' dormitory.

''Daphne,'' she said, moved to speak by the vision of Skip lying so weak in the hospital. ''I'm so worried about you and Skip. You know, he may not get better this time. He's so tired and so weak. And even if he does, it just doesn't seem possible that he'll ever have a job.

''And he could keep getting sick. Just like now. There's no way that you could work and take care of him, too. It would be too much for any one person.

''And no one knows whether he'll live very long. Even if he doesn't get sick again.

''And he'll never be able to have children.

''There're so many problems that face the two of you. I don't see how you two could ever make a life together.''

It was too much for Daphne. She could only nod her understanding. She was sick with worry about Skip. And now Patsy, in her quiet and loving way, was going down a future mother-in-law's checklist of problems.

Daphne felt a lump come to her throat and her eyes began to water. She was sure that only love prompted Patsy to say what she had said. That's the way Patsy was.

The meaning of the words was more than Daphne could bear. She managed to say goodnight without bursting into tears, but once inside the nurses'dorm, she sobbed uncontrollably. She had to see Skip again. She had to know that he was all right for tonight. She had to know that they were all right together. She had to hear him say that he wanted them to make it.

She borrowed a car and returned to the hospital and Skip's bedside.

She leaned down. He managed to raise his arms and let them rest around her shoulders. Daphne told Skip, between the sobs, about Patsy's conversation.

"Daph," he said, when she finished speaking. "We're going to make it. Look how far we've come already. Don't worry. Please. We're going to take it a day at a time. That's what we've promised each other. A day at a time. We knew it wouldn't be easy. But we're going to make it. The two of us. All of us."

She looked at him. He had been fighting a new round of sickness for weeks, yet he had enough still inside him to comfort her. She took a deep breath and began to dry her tears.

That night, when his life was again uncertain, Skip had found a reservoir of strength in his mother. Now he had shared some of that precious will and determination with the young woman he loved so deeply.

Three days had passed since I had been brought back to the hospital. It was February 11, 1971.

Dr. Poutasse was standing over me.

"Skip, I think we've found the cause of your problems. Your bladder, since our first operation, has begun to grow back some of that muscle. It can't empty completely.

"It's been continuing to hold some urine. Residual, we call it. And that residual has been creating serious infection. The antibiotics have been able to clear the infection each time we've used them, but they haven't eliminated the problem. We need to perform another resection. I've got to clip away some of that muscle that's grown back. You'll be on special medications from now on to prevent infection. But I think that will take care of it."

I never thought that I would be excited at the prospect of another operation, but I was. For the first time in nearly a month there appeared to be an answer. Something could be done to end the sickness.

I wondered to myself, when Dr. Poutasse left, "Could God have heard my cry to Him three days ago and allowed this answer to come?"

I really wasn't sure, but for the first time in my life I felt that maybe

God had answered me. In the only way that I knew how — quietly and alone — I thanked Him.

I was operated on the next morning. The second transurethral resection was simple and fast. Dr. Poutasse had cut away a little more muscle at the neck of my bladder. Once again my bladder began to function properly.

I bought an engagement ring while I was recuperating in the hospital.

One of my college friends dropped by to visit. He began telling me about breaking up with his fiancee. She had given the ring back to him. As he poured out his sorrows and fingered the ring absent-mindedly in his hands, he looked out the window toward the Elizabeth River.

"Skip, you know what I'm going to do when I leave here? I'm going to walk over to the river and toss this ring as far as I can."

I instantly thought how much I would like to have a ring for Daphne, but I knew that my finances wouldn't allow that for a long time to come.

"Hey, Larry, you can't do that. That thing cost a lot of money. I wish I had a ring . . ."

He looked up. "Here, you want this one? You can have it. I sure don't need it anymore."

"No," I said, "I couldn't do that." But I did become excited about the prospect.

"Here, take it." He shoved it toward me.

"No, I couldn't take it. What would Daphne think if she found out that I gave her a ring that somebody had just *given* to me?" I kept looking at that ring and thinking about Daphne.

He sensed that I wasn't going to accept it as a gift.

"Okay. Give me five bucks for it."

"Sold," I said.

I reached for my wallet, gave him five dollars and put the ring away. I didn't know when I would use it, but I definitely knew who was going to wear it.

I regained my strength, but I remained in Norfolk General for another operation. This one was scheduled for my hand.

Dad had followed up on the Albert Einstein test findings on my hands; there was a possibility for improved use of my fingers.

Before the bladder infection had sidetracked my life, I had visited with Dr. Jerome Adamson, a plastic surgeon in Norfolk.

I had no finger control in either hand. The little finger of my right hand was permanently extended, making it a constant and easy victim of cuts, scrapes and other damage. My other three fingers and thumb on my right hand were paralyzed in a folded position inside my palm. The fingers on my left hand also were folded into my palm. The best I could do was to use both hands as paws to pick up objects between them.

Based on examination and tests, Dr. Adamson believed that a successful tendon transplant could give me greater use of my fingers and hands. The transplant might provide some gripping ability to allow me to do things I could not do now. He decided to operate first on my right hand because it was stronger and had more potential than the left.

He explained that the surgery would be extremely long and complicated. Having fought the bladder problem, I was open to anything that might bring more improvement. I envisioned a normal hand after Dr. Adamson completed the operation, even though he cautioned me that that was not possible.

As I gradually moved from the darkness and sleep of the anesthetic in surgery into the light of my hospital room, I felt pain in my right arm. It was such a deep pain that I tried futilely to stay under the control of the drug. I looked at my right arm. It was attached to an IV pole and extended upright in the air. A cast encased my lower arm, wrist and my fingers to their tips. The throbbing ache reminded me of pain I had felt in my chest and my head only days earlier.

Dr. Adamson explained that scores of stitches had been required to close the surgery and that my arm should remain elevated, morning and night, for six weeks to allow it to heal properly.

The six weeks of recuperation at home were difficult for all of us. I was now unable to do anything for myself. I was helpless again. We constantly cheered each other with talk of my being able to use my right hand.

When Dr. Adamson cut away the cast six weeks later, I looked at an ugly misshapen and severely shriveled arm. The smell of the dead flesh and the dried blood and the sight of the endless lines of stitches made me faint.

I foolishly had expected a normal-looking hand. I didn't have it. But as I began to strengthen the atrophied arm muscles with prescribed exercises and to work with the fingers, I found that I did have some finger movement.

After the first operation, Dr. Adamson recommended a second operation on the hand. The thumb was not in its proper position and needed a pin to stabilize it. The tendon controlling the little finger needed to be tightened, and I needed more tendon work to allow me to lift my hand at the wrist.

The second hand operation in June was scheduled for six and a half hours, but was cut short. Some of the surgical work could not be performed. But the same pain was there when I came out of the anesthetic. And the cast. And the need to keep the arm elevated for six weeks.

When the second cast was cut away, I had some finger control and, because my thumb had been stabilized, I had some grip in my right hand. The fingers were still contorted, but not as badly as before the two operations.

A third operation was needed to complete the repair to my right hand. Then the same kind of operations would be performed on the left hand and fingers.

I couldn't bring myself to agree. And no one in the family tried to change my mind. I had endured the awful pain of surgery twice. I had some use of my fingers. I was willing to learn to live with that limitation, but I wasn't willing to go through another operation on my hand.

A reporter, Beth Polson, called me in March 1971 for an interview. She was the writer for the Lively Age section of the afternoon newspaper, *The Ledger-Star*.

The interview went well. She was easy to talk to and she showed an interest in me and my life. When I saw the interview in the paper, I felt a sense of pride and fulfillment for the family; someone had recognized how hard we had fought to keep going and was giving all of us credit.

She had asked two questions that, until the interview, I had avoided. As I read her interview, I was aware of how much she had helped me by forcing me to think about and to answer the two questions.

"What," she had asked, "do you plan to do when you leave Chesapeake Junior College this spring? And what are your goals in life?"

I hadn't thought about my future in terms that specific. But when she had asked, I had to come to grips with answers that satisfied me.

Now I was reading what she had written:

> "Everything to me is like a goal. I set small
> goals, then I set large goals."
>
> Among the large goals is an ambition to be
> a guidance counselor. "I'd like to come back
> here (Chesapeake College) to teach some
> day," he said. A psychology major, he plans
> to transfer eventually to Virginia Wesleyan.
> "We're not able to yet; it's too expensive," he
> said.
>
> Marriage is also among the goals. Right
> now he's dating a nursing student at DePaul
> Hospital.
>
> "I want to be a success," he said, "and
> help others in any way."

As I thought about what I had said in the interview — finish college, get a job and marry, I realized how badly I wanted to achieve those goals for myself, for Daphne and for the family. I knew that completing college was necessary to a life of security and independence and we had talked about it at home. But my special needs and the expense of college had raised a question that we hadn't yet answered: where to go?

The newspaper story helped us find the answer.

Three days after the story appeared, Dad got a call from Al Roosendaal, the father of one of my old football teammates. He was a member of a local Lions Club and he had read the newspaper story. He wanted to know if we might be agreeable to accepting financial aid from the Lions, if there were a college nearby where I could finish my education.

Dad had me in the car the next day, heading to Virginia Wesleyan College for an appointment with the president, Lambuth M. Clarke. I had heard good things about Wesleyan, but I hadn't visited there.

My first reaction to the campus was one of disappointment. Before Dad had parked the car, I could see problems. There were no ramps. I knew that there had been at least one wheelchair student. I wondered how he had gotten around. Some of the buildings were two and three stories high. That meant stairways. Were there elevators? The questions mounted as I glanced around the campus.

President Clarke's conversation erased many of the concerns. The buildings did have elevators. The college would schedule as many of my classes as possible on the ground-floor level. There would be no problems about transferring my credits from Chesapeake. My grades, he said as he reviewed them, were very acceptable and I would enter Wesleyan as a Junior.

The day after Mr. Roosendaal had received commitments from each of the Lions Clubs in the Virginia Beach area, he called Dad at home.

The Lions, he said, wanted to provide me with a scholarship to Virginia Wesleyan. It would cover completely tuition and books as long as I did my part and maintained a satisfactory grade level.

Suddenly the absence of ramps at Wesleyan was of no consequence to me. We had been given a way to provide for my continued education.

The gift from the Lions Club strengthened my belief that I could overcome whatever obstacles lay ahead. I wanted to finish school and I *was going to finish* school. That was the key to a job and a life with Daphne.

17

Our place at Carolina became our true summer home in 1971. Dad managed to acquire a larger trailer and he put it on a foundation next to Granny's and Papa's trailer. We had a growing number of guests. Karen was dating now and brought her friends to visit. The family spent every weekend there.

My hand was healing and my partial grip was becoming stronger as I pushed myself through my exercises. I was driven in part by a secret hope that perhaps I could find some way to return to my bass fishing. I often sat with Daphne on the lawn that bordered the Sound, watching bass fishermen heading out to work the grass beds and the shoreline.

Midway through the summer, on a warm, lazy Saturday afternoon, I held my fly rod in my hand for the first time in four years. Two friends, David Atkins and David Hopson, had helped me secure the rod in my right hand. We wrapped an elastic bandage around my open hand and fastened it at my wrist. I was able to slip the end of the rod between the bandage and my palm, using the new strength and flexibility in my fingers to steady the rod.

It felt comfortable and secure.

I began to try to cast the bug. I had little wrist movement and the first tries were awkward and unsuccessful. I kept at it and I was able to control the rod well enough to cast the bug in the direction I wanted it to land. It wasn't graceful, but it was effective.

The three of us got into the boat and headed for a near shoreline. David Hopson got out to fish alone. David Atkins checked my rod and bug and then tied the bow line around his waist. He began wading along the shore, working his rod and slowly pulling the boat. I was able to cast and suddenly I was bass fishing again.

We worked the shoreline all afternoon, finally giving up as darkness set in. I came home empty-handed, but I had improved my control over the rod and the bug.

My first bass since the accident came the next morning. It was small, not even a "keeper," but it represented another victory over my handicap. Landing the fish became a two-man job. When I felt the strike, I pulled back hard on the rod and hooked the fish, but I wasn't able to pull the line in with my left hand. I didn't have enough grip or strength. David came to the side of the boat and began taking up the slack in the line so I could play the fish with the rod. Slowly, as he continued to bring the line in, the bass came closer and closer to the boat. When it was beside the boat, I managed to grip the line and David raised the fish out of the water and into the boat. It didn't matter that the line had coiled around me and the chair. I had landed a bass.

As the summer neared its end, I was able to handle the line through my teeth and to play my fish without assistance.

I had found another reason to look forward to the future as we closed up the trailer for the winter. Bass fishing had become part of my life again.

Linda was married in the fall of 1971, just before I started at Virginia Wesleyan. I felt that I was losing touch with a very special person. In the spring, she had met Tom Viar, a student at the University of Virginia and one of the centers on the football team. They had dated steadily after their first meeting. I shared in her happiness but when she held me to say goodbye and to invite Daphne and me to visit her in Charlottesville, I felt that a large part of my life and my support was leaving. I realized how much she had done for me and just how much we loved each other.

Karen and her dates soon filled the void created by the departure of Linda and Tom. Shirley and I became closer and more attentive to each other now that we were frequently at home together.

My first day of classes at Wesleyan presented me with new problems. The college was much larger than Chesapeake Junior College and some of my classes had to be scheduled on the second floor.

I felt conspicuous as I pushed the button to the elevator to get to my second class of the day. I fumbled to get the key to the elevator into its slot. Nothing happened. I tried again and again. Still nothing happened. The elevator wasn't operating. I felt myself turning red with embarrassment as I realized that I was helpless and would be late for class on the first day. I wondered whether I would be able to handle this new environment.

My doubts ended as abruptly as they had started when a student offered to help. He stopped three others and the four of them lifted the chair and carried me up the stairs.

"I don't know how to thank you," I said as they put me down.

The student who had stopped to help me spoke.

"That's okay. There's a blind student here at Wesleyan, too. Carson Diggs. I help him out a lot in getting around and I read notes to him. If you need any more help, don't hesitate to ask. By the way, my name's Chuck Ratcliff."

I told him that I was uneasy about my first day at Wesleyan, I didn't know my way around, and it took me a long time to wheel from class to class — even if the elevators were working.

"Don't worry about it. I'll come back for you after this class and we'll get you where you need to go." With that, he turned and headed down the hall, leaving me with a feeling that I had found at least one student who understood some of my problems.

I had other adjustments to make. The first day of the second semester I was in a large class, larger than any I had ever attended. As I sat in the front of the room and students strolled in, chatting and kidding with each other, I again wondered if I could ever fit in at Wesleyan. It seemed so big and so impersonal.

The professor was late. When he came to the door, he announced in a terse voice that the class was being moved down the hall, that we were late starting, and that he expected everyone to move quickly to the new classroom.

Students began slapping their books in piles and shuffling out of the room.

I wanted to get started right away so I wouldn't be late, but I knew that I would cause a delay for the others. They filed out past me. There were no looks in my direction, no words spoken to me and no offers of help.

When the room was empty, I started pushing toward the new class. It was a long and frustrating push. The hallway was carpeted, which added to the problem. I wasn't adept at pushing the chair rapidly, even with the pegs on the rims. As I tried to go faster, my path became more and more erratic. It was a far cry from the run down the hall at Princess Anne, the day I started to run the hurdles.

A sense of anger at every student in the class began to build as I labored to get to the doorway where they had disappeared. The silence in the hallway was broken by the slamming of the classroom door. My anger grew into contempt. I didn't think anyone cared about me or my problems. There was no friendliness here, I thought. I conveniently ignored Chuck's help, the help of other students and the assistance of professors up until now.

I was five minutes late getting into the classroom. The professor and the class glanced up as I tried to open the door and push in. Someone helped me with the door and everyone quickly returned their attention to the lecture.

The pain of being ignored became greater than my bitterness.

"Why," I asked myself, "did no one help? What's wrong with them? What's wrong with me? How long is it going to be like this?"

I couldn't concentrate on the lecture going on in front of me. All during class, my mind kept repeating the questions. I tried to focus on the classwork, but it was futile.

I didn't get any answers to the questions. There was an answer, but I was too upset as I sat in class to remember it. Treacy O'Hanlan said it on the day I left Woodrow Wilson:

" . . . Be prepared to change for the world. Because it won't change for you. It doesn't owe you anything."

The awkward, zig-zag push down the hall that day taught me more about myself and what I would face than any course I had ever taken.

My requirements at Wesleyan began to lead me into an area of study that I hadn't anticipated. I was working for a degree in psychology in order to begin a career as a high school counselor. The psychology courses were supplemented with two required courses in religion. I had been raised in a Christian home and I had retained all of the information that my parents and our church had given me.

The religion courses began to raise questions. I began to have casual discussions with Mom about what I was learning of religions of the world. Initially, I think I was simply eager to show off, to let someone in the family know that I was being exposed to new and different views about religion and theology.

The knowledge that I acquired at Wesleyan triggered a torrent of doubts and questions. My religious background and my early lessons in church were being challenged. I didn't have the answers.

My discussions with Mom gradually grew into disagreements, then arguments. Some of my challenges to her beliefs were fostered by a change that I sensed in Dad. Before my accident, Dad had always spoken confidently of God and his faith in God; now he said very little. He continued to do things for me and the rest of the family, but he seemed to have doubts. He had been tireless in seeking medical help and any aid that would make my life more complete. The effort had caught up with him. He looked tired. Problems at work added extra pressure. He didn't talk much to us about his feelings. He kept everything bottled up until one of us would say something or do something that set him off. He'd sometimes react harshly and arguments and disagreements often resulted. He seemed to be lonely and unhappy. Yet I knew he was a Christian and his behavior puzzled me.

My arguments with Mom were more and more frequent. One afternoon, after a prolonged classroom discussion about Hinduism, I came home in an arrogant mood. I didn't have a faith and I felt that she had no valid reason for hers.

"Mom, how do you know that there's an eternal life with God? Who said so? And if you can't see God, how can you have faith in Him?"

She was insulted and she reacted angrily for a moment. Then she got out her Bible and began to show me Scriptures that supported her beliefs.

Her finger ran down the page until it rested on a verse in the Book of John:

> *"For God so loved the world that He gave His*
> *only begotten Son, that whosoever believeth in Him*
> *should not perish but have everlasting life."*

She calmed down and rested her argument as she watched my eyes follow the words. I couldn't understand how words on a piece of paper could bring such comfort to a person.

I found it more and more difficult to argue successfully with her. Her very reaction to my challenges and her response with Scriptures frustrated me. Her confidence in her faith made me want to have those same feelings, but I didn't know how to reach for them and I wasn't positive that I wanted to trade the way I was living my life for them, if that's what it took.

I didn't know what I believed in or what I stood for.

Shortly before Daphne's graduation from nursing school in June 1972, I talked with Dad about my plan to marry Daphne. As we talked and I shared my excitement about my future, I sensed that Dad might be trying to shake off some of the melancholy he seemed to feel and find a reason to look forward to the future. I thought that perhaps the knowledge that I was confident enough to talk about my marriage plans helped.

He didn't question our love for each other or the wisdom of getting married or where we would live or how we would support each other. His concern was more practical and fundamental. He was concerned only about my ability to continue to be covered by a hospitalization plan when I was no longer eligible under his policy. He knew the cost of hospitals and he knew that I was likely to find myself in one again for any of a thousand reasons. When he learned that the coverage could be converted to my name, he gave us his blessing.

Daphne and I hadn't settled on a wedding date, but her graduation prompted an exchange of important gifts.

She was to start a full-time job as an emergency-room nurse at General Hospital of Virginia Beach and she needed a car. She discussed the possibilities with me and told me that she wanted to buy a van because it would be more convenient for my travels. After the van was purchased, Mr. Via made a wooden ramp for the van, enabling me to be rolled in and out with ease.

It was only days after Daphne bought the van that I called and asked her to come to the house earlier than usual. She was expected for dinner, but I had something that I wanted to give her.

Any time we talked of an engagement, she said that she really didn't care about having a ring, and a ring wasn't important. I knew that she was thinking of me and the fact that I had only the money that the family gave me.

I watched from the living room window until she drove up to the house. I wheeled to my room and was making a pretense of serious study when she came in.

"Hi, hon. What're you studying?" she asked, kissing me and taking a chair beside mine.

"Not much of anything right now. I can't."

"Why?" she asked.

"Because I'm thinking of you. And us. Daph, are you sure you wouldn't like an engagement ring?"

"No, Skip. I've told you that before. Why would you ask me that?"

"Because this is for you," I said, extending my hand toward her and opening it. "I hope you'll like it."

Her expression was all that I could have asked for. She beamed.

"Oh, Skip. I love you so much! So very much. Where did you get it? How did you get it?"

The questions went unanswered as she hugged me.

18

Daphne and I sat close to each other as Tommy Viar's van rolled toward Elizabeth City, North Carolina. The date was September 23, 1972.

We were on our way to be married. We had decided to elope because Daphne didn't want to burden her parents with the expense of a wedding.

I reached frequently for Daphne's hand. Being able to touch and sense her presence helped me contain the excitement that had been building since I awoke that morning. We had talked often during the past two and a half years about a life together. We had planned and we had dreamed. I was surprised, now that our wedding day had arrived, that there was still excitement to be savored. Weeks earlier I had sensed the same excitement when Mom, Dad, Karen and Shirley worked with Daphne and me to ready a small refrigerator and some kitchen furniture for my room, which would be our first home. But it was nothing like the tingling sensation I felt now. Bubbling up inside me was a mixture of pride and happiness and excitement and a touch of apprehension.

After we bought our license, my feelings grew when I saw the church where Linda had been married to Tommy Viar the year before and where I was to be married now.

The day was September-perfect. A steady breeze moved the trees and the shrubbery in the churchyard. The sun shined down from a deep blue sky. Berea Baptist Church was a small, simple country church. It, too, seemed perfect for the ceremony.

Paul Bradley stood beside my chair as we waited for Daphne to come down the aisle with Tommy. Linda and Mary faced me on the opposite side of the aisle. A record of The Wedding March was playing.

Daphne appeared at the far end of the aisle. She was more beautiful than I had ever seen her, more beautiful than any woman I had ever seen.

We clasped hands and looked at each other as the minister started the ceremony. I tried to listen to all of the words, but I could only look at her and think how fortunate I was.

The minister had turned to her.

"Do you, Daphne Elizabeth Via, take this man, Alfred Thomas Wilkins Jr., To be your lawful wedded husband . . ."

Husband. The word *husband.*

I heard the rest of the words he spoke and I remember thinking briefly that I was sitting in a wheelchair when he said, ''in sickness and in health.''

He had ended his question.

Daphne squeezed my hand hard and smiled down at me in a way that I would never forget.

''I do,'' she said. Her voice was so soft and yet so clear and proud.

I had never known the feeling of such joy.

Our wedding-day breakfast was really an early lunch at a hamburger stand on the way back to Virginia Beach.

When we arrived at home, we were taken, accompanied by much fanfare from the family, to our new home. My room had been changed. Mom and Dad had given us their double bed, we had a small dining table and chairs, and furniture had been moved around to accommodate the small refrigerator that Daphne and I had bought.

We drove to the Vias and told them about our marriage. After their surprise subsided and the breathless questions of ''when'' and ''where'' and ''how'' were answered, they overwhelmed us with affection and wishes for happiness.

After dinner we all gathered in the living room. The conversation seemed endless and I kept looking at Daphne, wondering if it would be impolite to excuse ourselves.

Although we could not take a honeymoon trip because of finances and my classes, we were ready to begin our first night together. Finally the conversations ended and we went to our apartment. I was as nervous as any bridegroom must be on his wedding night and I had an apprehension that many never know. I could respond only to direct physical stimulation and often, doctors had warned, even that would be difficult or unsuccessful.

Whether it was Daphne's medical background or our long discussions about my limitations or simply the fact that we loved each other so much, our first night together as man and wife had all the completeness, all the tenderness, and all of the emotion that any man and woman could have. She helped me erase any apprehensions I had about my paralysis and my physical ability to make love and to be loved.

Later I put my arms around her and she fell asleep. As I looked at her beside me in the dark quietness of our room, I had but one thought: how happy and how whole, emotionally and physically, the woman I was holding had made me feel. I hoped that I had given her, that night, the same happiness.

Our life fell into a pattern dictated by Daphne's job and my classes. I was at Wesleyan until 11:30 some mornings and 1:30 in the afternoons the rest of the week. Daphne worked in the emergency room at Beach General on the 3 to 11 night shift. She worked every other weekend. Our home life centered around lunchtime meals. Mom provided my dinners and helped me prepare for bed when Daphne worked. Our social life centered on high school sports activities. Karen was still a cheer-leader and Shirley had become one, too. I took a lot of pride in them, especially Shirley, because I had encouraged her in her constant prac-tices to make the squad. On some weekends, when Daphne was off, we'd go out to dinner with Karen and one of her boyfriends.

My proposed topic for my senior project had been approved. I was doing a comparative study of individuals' personal interests before and after suffering traumatic injuries. Most of my research was done at Woodrow Wilson and Daphne and I spent many weekends with Linda and Tommy at their apartment in nearby Charlottesville.

In March I learned that the Community Mental Health Center in Norfolk was planning to open an adolescent daycare center and was interviewing for a part-time case aide. The idea of a job that could fit into my schedule at school and that was in the field that I wanted to enter excited Daphne and me. But the problem of transportation appeared to be too big to solve.

I mentioned the possibility of the job to one of our friends, David Terry.

"That's great, Skip," he said. "If you get the job, I'd be willing to give you a ride to work." David worked at a large grocery store on the same street as the planned daycare center.

I pursued the job and was selected. My first paycheck was for

$45.23. The check wasn't a lot of money, but it was another boost to my confidence. It also provided an opportunity for Daphne and me to take Mom, Dad, Shirley and Karen out to dinner.

As we chatted during dinner about the progress we had all made, I was sure that Dad was beginning to feel better about me, about my future and about himself. He was beginning to share his thoughts and his feelings again with the rest of the family.

In late April our routine suddenly changed. I had decided to stay home from Wesleyan because I didn't feel well. Daphne had left in the morning for a nurses' meeting.

I had become sensitive to the slightest change in my body's behavior and I was getting signals that something was wrong. My heartbeat began increasing. I became slightly nauseous and felt slight chills.

I knew what to look for and I found it. Once again blood was in my urine. David arrived, saw that I was sick and offered his help. Within hours, David, Mom and I were headed to Norfolk General Hospital in David's car.

Daphne arrived at the hospital shortly after Dr. Poutasse admitted me. I had left her a note when I couldn't reach her by phone at her meeting.

The next morning the X-rays pinpointed the reason for the latest sickness: both ureters, the tubes that carry urine from the kidneys to the bladder, were badly swollen.

Tommy and Patsy knew the scene all too well. For Daphne, it was her first experience in dealing with her husband's doctor and the onset of an illness.

Dr. Poutasse met with them in the hallway outside Skip's room.

"We've got a very serious problem this time," he said.

"I want to try a suprapubic on him first. It's a relatively uncomplicated procedure. A small incision above the pubic area directly into the bladder. The catheter's inserted in the incision.

"But you should know," he cautioned, "that Skip may very well face a major operation down the road. If the suprapubic doesn't work, we're looking at the need to bypass the bladder altogether. Medically, the operation is called an ileal conduit. What it means is that we will have to construct surgically a small reservoir from a piece of his ileum, that's part of his intestine, and the kidneys will empty into that. It will require an opening in his side and the need for a drainage bag on his side.

"But let's hope that we can avoid that."

When Dr. Poutasse came into my room, I knew immediately that he was concerned. We had been through so many crises together that we had come to know each other well.

"Skip," he said, "we've got some trouble this time. A TUR isn't going to get us through this one. Your bladder is stretched so badly that it can't function. The urine is backing up well into the kidneys and they aren't able to drain. We have to get them to drain."

"No TUR," I thought, "then, what?" My mind was reeling at the thought of what might have to be done.

"How?" I asked. "What . . . has to be done?" I really didn't want to hear the answer.

"I want to try a suprapubic. That requires a catheter inserted directly into the bladder right above the pubic area. We won't go through the penis again."

"No. No. There's got be something else. I'm married. I can't do it."

"Skip. Skip, just take it easy." He knew that I was agitated and his voice became soothing.

"We've got to do it. And I can't guarantee that this will work. But if it does, you don't have to worry about sex. Or anything else. It'll be less of a problem all the way around. Think about it. And take it easy. I'll see you tomorrow."

As the door shut, I closed my eyes. I didn't want another operation of any kind. I didn't want to be in the hospital. I wanted to leave. To go home and be with Daphne.

He hadn't told me what would happen if this new operation wasn't successful. But I knew. I had heard it called an ileostomy at Fishers-ville. The thought of it made me cringe. A bag attached to my side, constantly filling and needing to be emptied by someone because I couldn't use my hands that well. That and pressure sores were the biggest horrors for a quadriplegic. Each destroyed whatever dignity was left. Especially the bag. The need to have someone always empty it. And it could leak. Or break.

Mom came in.

"It's going to be all right," she said.

"No, Mom, I can't have it done. Not since being married. It's only been six months. I can't."

"Skip," her voice was firm, "if this has to be done, you'll have to have it done. Daphne knows. Dr. Poutasse has talked to her. She under-stands and she agrees with him."

"No." I was angry. "Please just leave me alone."

As she retreated to the door, I glanced down at the bed-bag, now half filled with red-tinted urine, reminding me of the problem.

I was thinking about the operation, trying to visualize the tube protruding from a hole in my stomach, when Daphne came in.

She didn't say anything; she just looked at me. Always, when she looked at me, I wanted to be strong and make her proud. This time it was hard to do.

"Daph, did he tell you what they want to do to me?"

"Yes, he told me. But don't worry. It's going to work. It will be better for us to live with. I know something about it."

"Are you just saying that? Do you really believe that? I don't know, Daph."

"I believe it, Skip. Just think. No more problems. No more wor-rying about when you'll get sick again. No more difficulty with your kidneys draining. It's going to be so much better."

Her acceptance of what was going to be done helped. If she believed things would be better, then I had to believe, too.

I had the operation on May 1. That night the blood started to clear from my urine. Two days later I went home. Dr. Poutasse told me that he would run tests on me in August to check the condition of my bladder. I was able to push the thought of a bag, always taped over the drainage opening in my side, out of my mind.

Wayne Whitley had joined Daphne and me for my last trip to Fishersville. I was headed to Woodrow Wilson for a final conference on the data I had collected for my senior project and I was going to take part in a bowling and pool-shooting exhibition by the disabled, all at Woodrow Wilson. The exhibition was new to me and I had decided to enter since I had to be at the center anyway. In addition, I had gotten pretty good at bowling with Daphne since my final hand operation and I still spent time shooting pool with the friends that came to visit us.

When I reported to the center early that Saturday morning for the competition, I was told to check in with the doctor.

"Why?" I asked.

"You need to be classified." I was told.

The doctor put me through the same series of tests I had undergone so frequently during hospital stays. He tested my reflexes, my muscle control, and the degree of paralysis throughout my body. I paid little attention when the doctor finally told me that I would participate as a "1A."

The bowling was as relaxing as bowling with Daphne at our local bowling alley. It didn't seem like an athletic event. And the pool-shooting was as enjoyable as shooting pool in the garage.

At the end of the weekend's events, I was awarded a first place in bowling and a second place in pool. Daphne was more excited about the medals than I was. I was impressed, however, with what I had heard about the track and field competition that had been held for the disabled. When we returned home, she hung the two medals in our apartment.

On my return from Fishersville, I made the last corrections and changes in my thesis and submitted it to my psychology professor. I began sorting my notes and studying for final exams. My grades were above the requirements needed to graduate and I wanted to end my college career on the highest note I could reach.

Several days later I sat outside the administration building waiting for graduation practice to begin. I would be the first person in the Wilkins family to graduate from college. I thought back over the problems and successes of the past five years. Two workmen began building a ramp to the platform as I watched. I knew that the ramp was for me. I thought of the pride that my diploma would bring to the family. Dad had worked tirelessly to insure an education for me. Linda and Mom had driven me so many times to and from class. Shirley and Karen had copied and typed countless assignments for me. Daphne and her belief in our future had become the greatest reasons for a sense of pride.

The professor coordinating the rehearsal called for attention. He explained that those seniors receiving diplomas would walk onto the stage, accept their diplomas from President Clarke and return to their seats.

He explained that the seniors who would not receive diplomas because of incomplete grades would be recognized and would cross the stage and shake hands with President Clarke.

He began to call out the list of those who would receive diplomas. As he worked his way through the alphabet toward the W's, I could feel the anticipation building.

"Roy Preston White."

My name was next.

"Rex Victor Willard."

He had skipped my name.

I suddenly wondered if I'd been skipped because I hadn't completed the oral defense of my research paper before the faculty committee. I had been late with my paper because I'd been in the hospital. I couldn't remember if my psychology professor had said anything about the orals. I didn't think he had.

The professor in charge of rehearsal began to call out the list of seniors who would be recognized, but who would not receive diplomas.

My name was on that list.

I located one of my professors.

It was the orals. I would have an incomplete grade until I presented my defense of my research. I could make the arrangements immediately after graduation and my diploma would be mailed to me.

I was dumbfounded. Not graduate? No diploma? How could I face anyone in the family? I rolled away from the practice and fought back tears. The thought of having to tell Mom was the pain that I felt now.

She was coming from the car to help me down the hill. She knew something was wrong.

"Skip, are you sick?"

"No, Mom. I'm not sick. It's worse. I'm not going to graduate with the rest of my class."

Patsy Wilkins was in shock at the words her son had just uttered. But the shock quickly left.

"What!" It wasn't a question. It was an exclamation. "What!" Then the question. "Why?" She was getting angry.

"Mom, I can't get my diploma because I haven't done my orals on my paper. I didn't know that. I can go through the ceremony, but I won't get my diploma until later."

Patsy thought of how Tommy would take the news. He was so proud that Skip was going to graduate. As were the girls. And Daphne.

"There's a mistake. There must be. I'm sure of it. I'm going to straighten this out right now. I'm going to see somebody. Where's the office?"

She was already headed toward the administration building as Skip called to her.

"No, Mom. Please don't. Forget it. Let's just go."

She continued her march, composing herself only after she'd entered the building and stated her mission to a receptionist.

The meeting had been civil, but just barely so, as far as Patsy was concerned.

She didn't talk with Skip on the drive home. She was trying to remember what had been said in the office to which she had been directed. She wanted to give an accurate report to her husband.

She hadn't lost her anger when she entered the office; she'd only managed to control it.

As well as she could remember, she had repeated what she had been told by her son.

The man behind the desk, in turn, had carefully explained the requirements for the senior project and the obligation of each student to schedule and complete an oral defense of the paper.

She tried to be precise in her recollection of the conversation:

"I understand that, sir. But my son was sick for more than a week. Can't he take the examinations now? Before graduation? We've worked so hard for this. All of us. Isn't there someway he can?" She bit her lip and maintained her composure.

"Mrs. Wilkins, I'm terribly sorry. I am. But we have to operate with certain requirements. They apply to everyone."

Patsy's anger grew.

"I can't believe that. He's met every requirement. Except this oral thing. He's worked hard. He deserves to graduate with his class. It means so much to him. To all of us."

The response was firm, and it was modulated to calm what the college official sensed was a distraught parent.

"Mrs. Wilkins, I'm sorry. We cannot change the rules. Your son has never asked special consideration since he's been here. We have to operate Virginia Wesleyan College with rules that apply equally to everyone. I cannot make an exception in your son's case. Please try to keep in mind that he will receive his diploma as soon as he has completed his oral defense of his paper."

"No!" Patsy spoke as if she were in command of the situation.

She wasn't exactly sure what the man had said then; she had lost her self-control. She thought she had heard something about "adjust to things," but she couldn't be sure.

"Adjust to things." Her mind was a whirl of scenes with Skip. The seemingly endless sicknesses. The constant caring for him. The lifting of his body to and from the bathrooms and tubs. The changes made in the house. The driving to and from school.

"Adjust? What does he think we've been doing?" she asked herself.

She had prayed hard not to give in to her impulse. She wanted to lash out.

She had looked one final time at the man behind the desk.

She then turned and strode out, not bothering to shut the door as she left.

The family was crushed at the news about graduation. I was embarrassed about not completing my oral defense on time and I was hurt because the family had been hurt. I couldn't bring myself to attend the graduation ceremonies. I went through my oral defense three days after the ceremony and passed without difficulty.

We weren't able to put the incident out of our minds until my diploma arrived in the mail. Mom was still hurt, but the receipt of the diploma began to mellow the rest of the family's feelings. I had, after all, graduated from college. And there was good reason to celebrate. Our pride wasn't shared with the hundreds of other students and families who had attended the ceremony at Wesleyan, but within our home, it was just as genuine.

I accepted a full-time job as a counselor at the daycare center. David continued to be my source of transportation as he still worked at the grocery store. I knew that many of my fellow classmates were still looking for work. It was with some surprise to me that I began to look back on my two years at Wesleyan with real appreciation. The professors had been good. They had worked with me and helped me deal with some of my inabilities. A number of the students had become friends. I had a solid college education. I had become genuinely interested in understanding more about religion. And I had made it on my own. I had a right to be proud of myself.

August came and with it my appointment with Dr. Poutasse for an examination to determine whether or not my bladder had returned to its normal size.

I had been feeling great all summer and there had been no problem with the suprapubic. But the thought of another IVP and what the results could mean brought back the worry of what could happen. I began to handle the fear differently. I prayed. I wasn't confident that God was going to hear or answer my prayers because I wasn't sure of my relationship with Him. But I felt I needed a miracle to heal my bladder. I acknowledged that my relationship with God was weak, but I believed that He alone could help me.

The IVP had been completed and I was lying on the X-ray table waiting for Dr. Poutasse to tell me the results. I was trying to decide how to express my gratitude if the X-rays revealed that I wouldn't have to have the operation that I feared the most: the ileal conduit. From somewhere, I had developed enough faith that God would help me through this to wonder about how to respond to Him.

"God," I prayed. "If everything turns out all right, I'll praise You right here."

Dr. Poutasse came in, carrying two X-rays.

"Skip," he said, "I can't believe this. Your kidneys have returned to normal size again. It is incredible."

Before he could show me the pictures or say another word, I said in a loud, strong voice, "Praise the Lord."

"You can say that again. There is no way that this should have happened. Do you know how close you were to serious kidney disease?"

It didn't matter how close I had been. The operation had been avoided. I had prayed to God as well as I knew how and my prayers were answered.

While the miracle of my healed bladder and kidneys gave Daphne and me cause for rejoicing, many of the little details of our life began to irritate me. Daphne had taken a new job and was driving me to work. My dependence on her began to bother me. I was often impatient with her when she helped me to dress in the morning. My temper flared more often than it ever had.

An argument about dinner one night climaxed when I slammed my fist to the table, causing a dish to fall to the floor and shatter.

Daphne broke into tears. She sat helpless and crying at the table. I wheeled out of the house to calm down. I couldn't understand why I had behaved in such a way. It wasn't my nature, yet it was as though there were some force inside me that compelled me to become angry and to hurt her.

Still without an answer as to why I had become so enraged, I returned to her and apologized as sincerely as I could. I told her that it wouldn't happen again, but I wasn't sure I could live up to that promise. I didn't know what was happening to me, but I wanted to find the answer.

I was on a roller coaster for the next few months. My temper would subside, then erupt. I had doubts about my future and what I should do with my life. I clung to the miracle that had happened in the X-ray room. It gave me at times the strength and the courage to suppress the doubts about my life and the guilt of my arguments with Daphne and others.

I began to realize that some of my troubled feelings came from the frustration of being able to do little for myself. Daphne took care of me almost totally. I had been building up resentment because I couldn't help myself, much less do things for my wife.

Slowly I began to bring my temper under better control and I ceased to become frustrated over little things that I couldn't do for myself. But I was lacking peace. I didn't feel that my life was being lived as fully as it could be.

Over and over I analyzed my circumstances. Physically, I was healthy. More importantly, I had no apprehensions about my medical future, now that the bladder problem apparently had been solved. My goals, the ones I had stated so long ago in a newspaper interview, had been achieved. I had worked hard and earned a college education. I was married. I had a full-time job. But something was missing.

Each time that I thought about my life and searched for an answer, I found myself thinking of Christianity and what I had learned about it from my studies and reading, from my parents and from Sunday School and church: a belief in God and in His Son. His Son died on a cross for me and for my sins, great and small. He promised eternal life. I had read these things. But I had never committed myself to such a belief. As a child I had been brought up to believe, but as a teen-ager and as an adult, I called on God only when I desperately needed Him. I always felt that I would be required to give up something in return for His help. I didn't like the idea.

My attitude gradually shifted from the doubts to a hope that perhaps Christianity was the answer that would bring me peace and a full life. The thought became constant during the fall and into the last months of 1973.

I had no major crisis. There was no single dramatic incident that led me. It happened one night at home with Daphne. I told her that I was going to set aside all my doubts and fears and that I was going to ask for forgiveness and the help of Christ. I realized that never before had I asked forgiveness or sought a purpose to my life. Help, yes. But not forgiveness. Not purpose.

I prayed that night in our bedroom. No bells rang. No light flashed. No cannon sounded. Something more telling happened. I sensed deep within myself that for the first time in my life I was being honest with God and with myself. I needed help; but more than that, I needed forgiveness.

That night I felt that a great weight, that had pressed down on me for so long, was lifted from my shoulders. I experienced an inner peace that I had never known.

As I closed my eyes for sleep to come, I acknowledged that God and His mercy had not changed, but that I had changed.

Part Three

19

The trip to Fishersville, Virginia, in May 1974, marked two more changes in my life.

Before Linda, Tommy and Daphne got into the car, they helped me into the driver's seat. I was a licensed driver. Dad and Jimmy Adkins, David's father and a family friend who had been helpful through the years, had installed hand controls in a 1969 Buick Electra, a gift from my uncle, Cle Wilkins.

We were headed to Fishersville where I would participate in competitive track and field events in the Virginia Wheelchair Games. I had received a registration form in the mail because of my participation the year before in exhibition bowling and pool. After looking over the forms, I had decided to enter the shot put, 40-yard dash, slalom race which was an obstacle course for wheelchair athletes, and table tennis. All for the first time. I'd played a little table tennis with the youngsters at the daycare center and with friends since the accident and I had heard about the track and field competition when I had last visited Woodrow Wilson. But that was all I knew of what was in store for me.

When the competition began early Saturday morning, I experienced feelings that I thought would never be possible again for me. The same sense of exhilaration that I had known in my high school athletics came back to me. There was constant activity on the field and I was fascinated by the varied techniques and forms of the others in wheelchairs as they limbered up.

Another emotion, one that I remembered only vaguely, came back as I rolled into the throwing circle. My heart beat faster and I had the same churning stomach that always had been there before the gun sounded in a race or before the opening kickoff in a football game. The shot was awkward and I had a difficult time trying to balance it for the first throw. When it landed, the small crowd that had gathered to watch the competition responded with applause and shouts.

I didn't know how far I had thrown, but the fact that I had been able to throw and the crowd reaction were rewards enough. I made my last two throws and left the circle. The official told me that I was in first place going into the finals later in the day.

In the finals, I improved with each of my three throws. I was overwhelmed when the official told me that I had unofficially broken a national record, as well as winning the event. As I signed the record sheet, the official asked me if I planned to compete in the national games in June. I had never heard of them, but I was encouraged by Linda and Tommy and Daphne who were as excited as I was.

"Yes, I guess so. I'd like to. What do I have to do?" I asked.

He explained that registration forms would be available the next day for the June national games in Washington.

In the hotel room, I rested between events, waiting for the table tennis competition. I kept remembering the scenes of the morning: the determination on the faces of the competitors; some of the athletes in colorful warmups; others, like me, in casual street clothes and tennis shoes; the officials who had been so helpful and encouraging to each competitor; the thrill of competing again and winning. I thanked God for allowing me to become excited again about athletics.

That night I added another victory to my first venture into competitive wheelchair sports when I won the table tennis event. Daphne and I rushed to a telephone to tell Mom and Dad about my performances. They were as happy as we were and they assured me that the whole family would drive up to Washington to see me compete in the national games.

As the excitement of the day ebbed, Linda, Daphne and I talked quietly in the hotel room.

"Linda," I said, "for the first time in my life I had a peace with God."

"You know, Skip, I prayed and accepted God right after your accident, but sometimes I still have doubts."

"I know. So do I. But I think that's normal. What is most important is that we know in our hearts what we believe."

Daphne had been quiet, listening to us. Linda turned to her.

"What about you, Daph, are you a Christian?"

She was startled. "I guess so. I've gone to church."

"But have you ever asked God into your heart? Have you been saved?" Linda asked.

"I don't know about things like that. I don't think I'm a bad person the way I am now."

The three of us, in an earnest and naive way, began to talk about salvation as we understood it, seeking answers to our questions in a Gideon Bible that had been on the night table. The Bible listed a series of questions about a Christian life and cited Scriptures in providing the answers.

We talked a long time. Finally Daphne turned to me.

"Well, I need salvation because I want to be in Heaven with you, Skip. What should I do?"

We turned again to the Bible and read aloud the steps that were outlined. The three of us then closed our eyes and Daphne said a prayer, asking for forgiveness and salvation. I was moved very much by what had happened and I was happy for Daphne because of my own experience.

Linda left to rejoin Tommy in their room.

Daphne talked for awhile.

"I don't feel any different, Skip. Am I supposed to? I do know that what I just did feels right."

"Let's just take it slowly," I responded, "like I've been doing. "Like we've been doing. A step at a time."

That night, we prayed together. It was a short prayer and perhaps awkwardly worded, but it was a prayer offered for the first time by the two of us as husband and wife.

A door leading back to athletics and a door leading to a Christian family life opened to us on that 1974 return to Woodrow Wilson.

On our drive home I received a disappointing lesson in geography. Daphne was reading the registration forms for the national games as we headed back to Virginia Beach. The nationals would be held in Cheney in Washington State, not Washington, D.C., as I had assumed and as I had told Dad on the phone.

It was a blow. "That's all-the-way-on-the-West-Coast Washington," I sighed. "We can't go there. It would cost a fortune."

Beth Polson and her newspaper, however, helped us overcome the problems of distance and dollars. She wrote a story about my performance at Fishersville and my interest in going to the nationals in the state of Washington. Individuals and businessmen responded to the story with financial contributions. I opened a travel account and Ran Randolph, a vice president at the bank, became interested in me and began to help me with the accounting.

Before I left for the West Coast, Karen received her diploma from Princess Anne. It served as another reminder, as we celebrated, of how close we were as a family.

Daphne and I boarded the plane for Spokane, Washington, on June 14, 1974. Neither of us had traveled such a distance from home and we wondered what we would find when we landed on the West Coast. We had packed every item that I would possibly need. In some cases, we carried two similar items each in a different bag in case one bag was lost. The last item that I put in the suitcase was my Bible. Daily, I spent a quiet time reading and studying.

The pleasure of traveling together to a new place was rapidly giving way to fatigue and the shock of changing time zones when Daphne pulled the rental car into a parking space at Eastern Washington University, the site of the games. Daphne rolled my chair to me and I noticed that my cushion wasn't in the chair. I had reminded her about the cushion when I had transferred from the chair into the car at the airport. I had last seen it resting on the rear of the car before we pulled away.

"Daphne, where is the cushion?" I asked.

She was quick to respond.

"Haven't you got it? I thought you picked it up before we left the airport."

I lost my temper. "You better have it. Or you better find it. I told you to take care of it." I was scared. The idea of sitting for any length of time, much less competing, without the cushion was alarming. It was as much a requirement to meet my basic needs as water and food. It was part of an arsenal of special equipment; it helped prevent pressure sores. I became angry enough to want to strike out at something. So I did. I rammed my elbow into the car door. Hard. Then again. I completely lost control of myself. Daphne was close to tears. I was embarrassed at my childish reaction to the missing cushion and my elbow was aching, but neither feeling erased the fear of sitting for days without a cushion.

We drove back to the airport, searched the area where we had picked up the car, and inquired inside the terminal. No cushion.

We were exhausted. It was 2 a.m. on the West Coast and 5 a.m.

back home. We didn't know where our room was and we couldn't find anyone awake at the college. Daphne's tears finally came. Someone eventually helped us find a vacant room. We had been up for nearly 24 hours. But the beds, typical of some college dorms, were only a foot or so high. I didn't think that I could successfully transfer into one of them. And if I could, I wondered how I would get out. We called Dad who said that he would put another cushion on a plane that morning.

We finally managed to lie down. We were tired and frustrated. This wasn't what I had envisioned when the official back in Virginia had asked me if I planned to compete in the national games. I didn't even pray. I was simply and totally defeated.

The morning, after a little sleep, brought our promise to each other that we would make the best of our situation. We both prayed. I asked forgiveness for my actions and we prayed for the safe arrival of the second cushion and the strength to pull ourselves together.

When we registered, we were moved into a room with higher beds. We began to meet a number of athletes and we studied the schedule of events.

I had developed a small open wound on my rear from sitting so long without the cushion the night before. Daphne suggested that I continue to lie down that afternoon and rest while she drove to the airport to get the second cushion.

She remained away for a long time and when she finally returned, I could tell from her expression that there was no cushion. I lashed at her again. She had looked everywhere at the airport for the cushion. She had even started back to the baggage claim area, but the airline agent had told her that he had checked and it wasn't there.

I rode with her as she drove for the third time to the terminal.

In the baggage claim area, slowly making its circular journey on the conveyor belt, was the cushion.

Again that night we tried to calm ourselves, but my prayers became questions about why we were being confronted with only problems. I couldn't understand why God would make this experience so difficult after all that I had been through.

There was another worry the next day as competition began. The heat was intense, sapping my strength and making me dizzy. I lost in the third round of table tennis and had to struggle to win the consolation match and a bronze medal.

I faced the same kind of heat the following day. Daphne was my only ally. She was my trainer, my coach and my cheerleader. She tried to cool me down with ice packs on my head and my neck between events. At the end of the day's trials in the field events, I knew that it wasn't going to be like my entry into wheelchair sports back in Fishersville. I was out of the running in the slalom. I did, however, hold first place in the shot put trials.

Daphne and I relaxed for the first time the night before the finals. We had been through a tough time on our first trip together. The experience had been so unpleasant that I questioned whether winning a first place — still a possibility in the shot — would make up for all the heartache.

I was denied the victory. I remained in first place until the next-to-last competitor's name was called — Rod Vleiger, who had beaten me in table tennis. On his last attempt, he bettered my mark. I was next up and, despite the best effort I could give, I didn't overtake him. I was awarded the silver.

Daphne knew that I was depressed as we headed for the room after the meet. She tried to bolster my spirits.

"You shouldn't feel so badly, Skip. It's only your first year. I think you really did well."

"I know it's my first year. But I wanted to win. This trip has been terrible. You haven't had any fun. Neither have I. I've had all the traveling that I ever want to do. I just want to go home."

I was defeated physically, emotionally and spiritually. The two medals that I had won weren't enough to remove the bitter taste of defeat and dejection as we headed back to the East Coast and home.

Our misadventures and my defeats in Washington received a variety of antidotes when we got home.

Physically, my biggest concern was the small wound that had opened on my posterior. I knew about pressure sores and what such sores could do, even in a nonathletic life. I was apprehensive when the doctor examined me. He told me that the wound wasn't on a pressure area and prescribed a medicated cream and confinement to bed for five days. The wound finally closed, leaving a calloused spot on my rear and a frequent worry in my mind because the callus didn't disappear.

Emotionally, Daphne and I had been out of control. But from the experience, we had learned a lot about ourselves under stress and we knew that we had to be on constant guard against striking out at each other for any reason. We had grown closer as a result of facing difficulties together, but we were aware that we had a lot to learn about communicating with each other and about living a Christian life together.

The deepest wound from the Washington trip was spiritual. I hadn't behaved in a Christian way. I had responded to minor problems with outrage. My faith had vanished when the circumstances became adverse. I began to understand that I had equated belief with the ability to say a prayer and to look for an answer. I began to look at the way I lived my whole life. What I saw wasn't pleasant. I needed to change my behavior. I began to realize that I couldn't pray for situations always to be pleasant, but that I could seek God's help in handling such situations in a different way. I recognized that I was weak and that I needed God's strength to help me change. I began to read the Bible more thoughtfully, seeking the Scripture that would help me change. I shared these feelings and these efforts with Daphne. Together, we began to feel good about ourselves and about my effort to learn more about God's desires for our lives.

There was a celebration at Carolina. Dad and Mike Preziotti completed work on a new bass boat for me. They had mounted the seat and backrest assembly of a wheelchair on a swiveled pedestal in the boat. The seat gave me the mobility to drive the boat from a secure position, reducing the possibility that I might fall over the side. The boat was 14 feet long with a 68-inch beam and a 50-horsepower motor mounted on the transom. Using the specially designed crane and pulley to board and leave the boat, I was now able to travel anywhere on the Sound in search of bass. The boat was fast enough to use for pulling skiers and I once again was part of the family's enjoyment of the water.

The boat, in that summer of 1974, fulfilled a hope that I had clung to for six years, since my first return to Carolina and the Sound in 1968.

My ability to drive a car and get around on my own and the stability of my job allowed Daphne and me to turn our thoughts to her professional needs. Her job with the Health Department in Norfolk was convenient, but it didn't offer the clinical work that she enjoyed so much. We decided to work toward a more personally rewarding job for her.

In addition to clinical and administrative opportunities, the job also had to offer day hours and weekends off so that we could be together as much as possible. We were determined that our family life always would be our first consideration.

Daphne took the required exams for nurses' openings in civil service and was placed on a hiring list.

Within two weeks, she received the offer of a position with an impressive increase in salary. The hours, however, called for night work and alternate weekend duty. We agonized over the decision and prayed for guidance. Finally, in spite of the tempting salary, she declined.

We wondered for days whether it had been the right decision. We continued to pray. The next telephone call she received was the offer of a position at the Norfolk Naval Air Station Dispensary. The days and hours were perfect, the salary was higher than the job she had declined, and she was able to ride to and from work with Dad, whose office was nearby on the Naval Base. In October 1974 Daphne returned to the kind of nursing practice that she most enjoyed.

I began to sense a confidence now that both of us were growing as Christians. We had faced a lot of problems, some big and some small. Some we handled well, with God's help. Other times we fell flat on our faces and had to pick ourselves up and begin again. But I knew that our lives had changed for the better, and I received an important piece of evidence soon after Daphne began her new job.

Angie Spruill worked with me at Community Mental Health. We talked frequently about the challenges of our jobs and constantly different counseling approaches needed for the individual children in our care. There was always pressure.

One day Angie asked me, ''Skip, how come you are handling the problems here so calmly? You seem to be different from the way you were when you first came to work.''

''It's all in God's hands, Angie. He's the One who guides me now.''

She wanted me to explain. As I began to talk about finding my faith, she shared her fears and her confusion.

"I've looked so long for the kind of peace that you have," she said.

With that brief conversation as a beginning, Angie and I began Bible study together. Another co-worker, Clara Paige, joined us. I felt that we were giving and receiving strength from each other and, in some way, doing God's work with Him.

The opportunity to touch more people came in February 1975, after a pleasant evening in my parents' home. Our pastor, Dick Woodward, and his wife were dinner guests. The family had started attending his church, Virginia Beach Community Chapel, in 1973. Dick Woodward had visited me in Norfolk General shortly after the accident and I had remembered his kindness and concern. Tabernacle Church, where Mom had received so much strength, was the mother church to Community Chapel.

During the after-dinner conversations, Dick Woodward became very interested in my feelings about the accident and how I had begun to find my faith. We talked for a long time.

Before he left, he asked, "Skip, would you mind sharing your life with others?"

I wasn't sure what he had in mind, but I said that I would be happy to do it. He said that he would like for me to speak to the congregation at a Sunday morning service.

I was flattered that he felt I had something to contribute, but I was also nervous. Nearly 700 people attended the Sunday service at Community Chapel.

My anxiety about speaking to a large group of people soon was mixed with the anticipation of sharing my life with so many others.

When I looked out over the congregation on that Sunday, I saw the faces of many people who had helped me and my family. It was comforting. I began to tell them the story.

I wasn't able to reflect much on my speaking when I went to the social hall after the service. Hundreds of people came to me and told me how much they appreciated what I had said and they told me that they had gained a stronger personal faith because of my story.

At home, I was able to think back on my talk. I was pleased that other people liked what I had said. More importantly, I was thankful that God wanted others to hear about my thoughts and my faith.

Several days later, Dick Woodward asked me to consider becoming the youth pastor at Community Chapel, helping to meet the spiritual needs of the young people in the congregation.

I was hesitant. "I don't know that much about the Bible and formal study. I'm still learning."

"I understand that, Skip," Dick responded. "We can teach you those things. If God wants you in this ministry, you will know."

I weighed the offer at Community Chapel. Tentatively at first and then with certainty, I came to the realization that I needed and wanted much more understanding of God's word. My initial response to Dick Woodward — "I don't know that much about the Bible" — became a goal of learning. There was no further discussion about the youth ministry and that possibility passed. But what was left was my feeling that God had given me a direction.

20

One path to a greater understanding of the Bible led me to a kind and mild-mannered man named Ozzie Pretzman. He was an active member of Community Chapel and had heard me ask for prayer about going into God's work at a Sunday School dinner. He asked to visit. The next morning, before I had gotten up, Ozzie was sitting at the foot of my bed, asking me about my life as a Christian and about my study of the Bible. His interest in me and his vast knowledge of the Bible made me realize that I had a growing faith in God, but that I didn't have a clear understanding of that faith or how to strengthen it.

He came to the point of his visit.

"Would you like to know more, Skip, that will help you understand and build your faith in God?"

I was eager to study with him. Before he left, he gave me two assignments. The first, he said, was the most important. It was to learn John 14:26. This, he said, was the key to begin Bible study. The second assignment was a two-lesson Bible study.

"Call me, Skip, if, and when, you are ready to take the first step," he said.

By the day's end, I had read, reread and memorized the verse from John:

> *"But the counselor, the Holy Spirit, whom the
> Father will send in my name, will teach you
> all things and will remind you of everything I
> have said to you."*

I had completed both of the study lessons. I not only was ready for the next meeting with Ozzie, I was eager.

By mid-April 1975 I was deeply involved with Ozzie in a study of the Word. Daphne had joined with me and together we marveled at the discoveries that we were making as we learned the Bible's messages.

Wayne Whitley called one evening to ask me to serve as a reference for him. He had learned that the City of Virginia Beach soon would open a short-term adolescent care facility; he wanted to apply for one of the counselor positions. He told me that the city was looking for a director and an assistant director. There were increasing problems at

Community Mental Health where I worked. Some involved funding and others involved the counseling programs. Wayne encouraged me to apply for one of the new positions. I barely met the application deadline for assistant director or chief counselor. I was told that a decision would be made within the next two weeks.

A few weeks later, heading toward Fishersville and the 1975 regional wheelchair meet, I thought back to the difficulties that Daphne and I had experienced in Washington in 1974. I hadn't been certain that I would ever travel or compete again after the trip to Cheney. But many people had encouraged me to keep trying. Bill Taylor, a local businessman and a friend through our Community Chapel activities, and his brother had offered to sponsor travel for Daphne and me to regional meets and the nationals, if I qualified. Martha Willey, who with her family owned a sporting goods store, had provided me with practice equipment — shot, javelin and discus, two new events for me — and warmup suits and shoes. Their support was added incentive to do well. My practices weren't very formal. I worked out in our front yard with Shirley providing encouragement and retrieving my throws. I won the shot, the discus, the javelin and table tennis at Fishersville and easily qualified for the nationals.

Mom and Dad had driven to Fishersville. It was the first time that they had seen me compete. Dad didn't say a lot at the end of the meet, but he had a smile that I hadn't seen in a long time. He had witnessed something that he hadn't thought would ever happen: my return to athletics. He was proud of the medals, but the fact that I was competing again was his greatest reward. His doubts about my future were finally gone and he had come back to us.

As I started pulling myself back up in the athletic world, my work world came crashing down on me and all of my colleagues. Each of us was called into the administrator's office in mid-May and told that the Community Mental Health program would be terminated at month's end. I was almost relieved at the news; conflicts and program problems had gotten out of hand. I had lost my job and I had no immediate prospects of another one, but I believed Daphne and I would survive the setback. I called Daphne, told her the news, and headed for Granny's and Papa's place at Carolina where I could think about the future.

That evening Daphne called. She was so excited that she hardly could get the words out. The administrator of the planned crisis intervention home for adolescents in Virginia Beach had called to explain that the staffing effort had fallen behind, but they now were ready to begin selecting employees. He wanted to know whether I was still interested in being interviewed. She relayed to him my very positive response and he set up an appointment.

Wayne appeared at Carolina the next morning. He had heard about my loss of a job and Daphne had suggested to him that I might enjoy his companionship. Wayne and I had drifted apart after my marriage and my settling into a family routine. The few days together, just the two of us fishing and remembering old times and talking about our lives, brought us close together again.

Wayne drove with me to my interview. Before the questions started, Bob Dunsmore, regional administrator for the program that would include the Crisis Home, explained to me that the operation of the home initially would not require an assistant director or a head counselor. He wanted to interview me for the director's position, based on my previous work, if I was interested in that. I quietly said a prayer that the wisdom and the experience I had gained would be sufficient for the job.

Near the end of the interview, he paused for a few moments.

"Skip," he said, "I'm very much impressed with your insight into young people and your knowledge of counseling. You've also got the kind of experience that I'm looking for to develop this program. I've got to ask you a tough question, but an obvious one, about your physical limitations."

He explained that the home would be quartered in a two-story building. Sleeping accommodations for some of the youngsters would be on the second floor.

"How would you get to the second floor when you are needed there?"

I didn't have an immediate solution, but I did have a response.

"If you feel that I can handle the unknown problems that will come up with the kids, I feel that I can find an answer to this problem that we both know exists."

It wasn't a direct answer to the question, but I truly believed that if this job were meant for me, I could find a solution. I was not going to be defeated because of a wheelchair.

Interviews with other candidates were to continue through the week. Four people would be selected for final interviews before a committee.

Wayne and I returned to Carolina. Two days later Daphne called.

"Skip, the Crisis Home called you for the group interview. You're going to get that job. I just know you are."

That night I thanked God for giving me the ability and the knowledge to progress with the interviews as far as I had.

The committee interview was exacting. Their questions covered everything from religion to drugs, from sex among teen-agers to a family's role in rearing children. I came away with a feeling that I had been responsive to the questions and had impressed the four members of the committee.

My feeling was confirmed the next evening as Wayne, Mike Preziotti, my long-time fishing friend, and I prepared to head out in the boat.

Granny hollered to me that Daphne was on the phone.

Daphne was almost breathless.

"Skip, you got the job. Mr. Dunsmore just called. He asked me to call you. You were the unanimous choice of the committee. You're the *director* of the Crisis Intervention Home."

I listened in near disbelief. I had known that I was reaching high in trying for the directorship of a brand new agency. And suddenly, I had grasped what I was reaching for. It took a moment for me to absorb what I had heard.

Daphne said that she would join me for the weekend as soon as she could, but that she wanted me to know right away how proud and how happy she was.

The national games in Champaign, Illinois, were scheduled to end only four days before I was to begin my job as director. The meet was vastly different from the nationals in Washington the year before. There was no lost cushion, no loss of temper and no angry words. My attitude was one of thankfulness that I was able to compete. Physically, I was better prepared for the events. At the end of the trials I was in first place in the shot, second in the javelin, and third in the discus. I made it into the finals of table tennis, but was defeated by Rod Vleiger, the same athlete who had beaten me the year before. I wanted a gold medal. I especially wanted to beat Rod in the shot. But I was more motivated by a desire to have a good attitude than by a desire for personal glory, thanks to my studies with Ozzie.

At the close of the final events, I had won two silver medals, one in the discus and one in the javelin. I had also won a medal in the shot. It was the gold. I had beaten Rod and had broken the national record that he had set the year before.

I was nominated for the U.S. team which would compete in Mexico. I wasn't selected, but I had done the best I could. That was satisfaction enough.

After the Washington meet, Daphne and I had almost given up; I had nearly quit athletics. Now I knew that I'd be back to compete in 1976 and that I had the same chance as anyone else did to make the U.S. team and to compete in world competition.

When I got home, I became totally absorbed in my new job. Many of the responsibilities of directing the Crisis Home, as it came into being, were new to me.

The home was designed to be a short-term residential facility for children who had not committed criminal offenses, but who were problems at home or in school. Repeated runaways, truants and similar troubled youngsters were to be in our care. The courts referred to them as "status offenders" and the home was to provide an alternative to the area detention homes, where many were being sent and where they had to mingle with true lawbreakers.

Our mission was to provide a "cooling off" period away from the cause of the problem. We were to try to open up communication with the children, provide counseling when it was warranted, and return them to their homes and classrooms after their particular crisis had passed.

I relied on guidance from Bob and his assistant, John Roberts, as I interviewed and hired a full staff and began to operate the home. I hired Wayne as one of the counselors, based on his past experiences at the juvenile detention home. The varied backgrounds and experiences of the staff gave me confidence that we could administer successfully to the young people who were sent to the home. From the outset, I tried to foster a work environment that allowed us to share our strengths and overcome our weaknesses as a cohesive group. It was not always easy or pleasant, but even in the early days of our work, we had a sense of openness and fellowship. The Virginia Department of Rehabilitation was a big help. Based on my employment and my limitations, the department provided a ramp to my office and a stair elevator to the second floor.

I had to appear frequently in court on behalf of some of our young wards and I had to visit other facilities affiliated with the city's juvenile program. The Department of Rehabilitation also was instrumental in helping me meet that need. Through its efforts, I purchased a van, and Mace Scientific, a local firm, outfitted it with an electronically operated sidedoor and wheelchair lift. I was able to get in and out of the van and to transfer from the wheelchair to the driver's seat without help. The final barrier to an independent life had fallen.

As the fall of 1975 arrived, I was responding almost solely to the demands of the Crisis Home. I spent long hours in the office dealing with daily problems and almost always would take administrative paperwork home. Soon we began to function at capacity and the home began to have a positive benefit to many of the young people who were sent there. All of us worked under steady pressure. Often I would receive calls late at night or early in the morning that required me to leave Daphne at home in order to stop a minor difficulty from becoming a major problem.

The pace tired me and left me little strength. The callus that I had tried to put out of my mind became irritated and then split open. Often during these weeks, I was able only to go to work and return to bed, as the doctor ordered, in an effort to heal the lesion. Without complaint, Daphne shouldered the responsibility for caring for me in addition to her job. Both of us found time in the evenings to continue to study the Bible and to discover what God's message to us was in this new set of trying circumstances.

The more disconcerting the problems became, the more I submersed myself in study and prayer. I met weekly with Wayne, Bud Hooper, a probation officer who worked with the Crisis Home, and Rob Ulsh, who was the youth director at Community Chapel. The four of us shared our experiences of trying to live Christian lives and we studied and discussed God's Word in the Bible and the books we had read that interpreted that Word.

From these weekly meetings I began to examine the role of fasting as a prayer of sacrifice to God. As the pressure of the job and the continual worry about the callus increased, I fasted; sometimes for a single meal, sometimes for a full day.

My three friends became a support outside the home as strong as Daphne and the family were inside the home. Daphne and I grew even closer in our thoughts and actions as we studied together and sought to understand why we always seemed to face adversity.

Despite my physical discomfort, I began in the spring of 1976 to prepare for the year's competition. Whenever I had a few spare minutes, I practiced in the lot next to the Crisis Home. One afternoon Wayne stopped to watch me. He began to offer some suggestions and to work with me. He had some excellent ideas. After several afternoons together, we agreed that he would work with me as often as our time permitted. I now had someone to help me, to watch my form, to correct me and to help me discover ways to improve. Most importantly, Wayne provided encouragement.

Wayne was with me, as were Daphne, Mom and Dad, as I performed at Fishersville. I don't know who was more rewarded by my performances: Dad, Wayne or me. I set national records in the shot and in two events that were new to me: the club throw and the precision club throw. In the first competition I threw a wooden club, similar in shape to a small bowling pin, for distance; the second competition was for accuracy as well as distance. I also won the discus and javelin.

My next meet was on Long Island in June. Once again, the possibility of being on the U.S. team for international competition loomed. My strong performances at Fishersville and the close relationship that Wayne and I were building almost daily prompted me to think from time to time about selection to the team, the goal of every wheelchair athlete.

I had learned a great deal about wheelchair sports since my beginning at the pool table and on the bowling lanes.

Regional competition was held each year in April and May at 15 locations throughout the United States. For many, participation in the regionals was a goal in itself. Just to be active, to be athletic again, was a reward to many of us who had been disabled.

Beyond the regional meets was the national competition. This was open to those who had met established performance standards in any one of the regional meets. The nationals were held once a year in June at a place selected by the National Wheelchair Athletic Association.

Selection by an NWAA committee to participate as a United States representative in international competition was based on over-all performance in the national meet. There were other criteria — the availability of housing and the availability of funds to cover the cost of the trip for the American athletes. Because the NWAA relied on contributions for the games, the size of the team varied from year to year. Sometimes as few as 25 athletes represented America; at other times the number swelled to 50 or more.

A series of letters back and forth from the NWAA before we left for Long Island lessened the prospect of being selected for the world games.

The first letter was from one of the U.S. team coaches. It contained information about the international Paralympics. It had a small typed postscript. The note asked whether I could take complete care of myself if I were selected for the international meet.

I responded that I would have no difficulty because my wife was a nurse and was accustomed to helping me with my needs.

A second letter from the coach advised me that the site for the games, Toronto, Canada, did not have facilities to accommodate husbands and wives. It stated in very simple language that I must be prepared to take complete care of myself without assistance. It went on to state that further discussions would be held in Long Island, if necessary.

It was the second letter that increased my determination to make the team even as it reduced the possibility. I compiled an inventory of the things that I could do for myself and the things that Daphne had to do for me. I began to design solutions to my dependence on Daphne for even the smallest needs in the event that I qualified and she couldn't stay with me.

The prelude to the actual competition in Long Island could not have been more positive. Two friends, Becky and J.K. Pell, had driven from Kentucky to be with me. Daphne and I had met Becky through Community Chapel at Virginia Beach. They had moved to Kentucky when

J.K. had gotten out of the Navy, but we continued to correspond. Wayne and Daphne were there. I had all the personal support I could ask. At the outset, however, it didn't appear that their presence and support would be enough. I lost my semifinal match in table tennis and managed only a third-place bronze at the end of the first day's competition. I had learned many things from my Bible study during the past months and I was able to talk peacefully with God, asking that He help me deal with my anxieties and allow me to concentrate on my attitude.

The table tennis defeat had been erased from my mind as I prepared for the field events the next day. I knew that I was ready to do my best. I won the shot put with the longest throw ever recorded in the United States by a 1A quadriplegic. Wayne's help had paid off and it was to pay off again. I won the javelin for the first time in my career and I took a silver in the discus.

Sy Bloom, the head U.S. coach who had written the letters to me before the games, had not mentioned the Paralympics to me during the entire meet. As we waited on the final evening for him to announce the names of the U.S. team, I was certain that my achievements had eclipsed any problem about living conditions and caring for myself.

No matter how many times Sy stood before the assembled athletes, their coaches and their friends and family on the final evening, the announcement of the members of the U.S. team was always fresh, always filled with drama and always the highest accolade that an athlete could receive. It was more than recognition by one's peers in that group of special — some would say different — athletes. It was a chance to represent our country before the world and to represent every person who is disabled. It was a chance to say, "This is what we can contribute when we are provided the opportunity."

Sy explained the team selection process as his yearly preamble to the announcement of the chosen athletes. I reached for Daphne's hand.

"Daph, whatever will be, will be. Right?"

She smiled back her acknowledgement and squeezed my hand.

The audience was quiet. As each name was called, there was applause and cheering. Then silence again. Then another name and applause. At the end, there had been no applause for my name; it hadn't been called.

I looked at Daphne, then Wayne.

Wayne managed a smile. "Next year," he said and winked.

Wayne was right. It would have to be next year. I was disappointed. But I truly believed that God did not have the Paralympics in His plan for me this year.

We left the banquet hall to pack.

Just before we headed for the highway and home, we made a final stop at the hall for ice for soft drinks in a cooler.

I was amazed when Wayne came out and told me that several of the athletes were arguing with Coach Bloom about not putting me on the team.

I wanted to let him know that I hadn't initiated the lobbying effort. When I got inside, the discussion had cooled down and I had an opportunity to introduce myself to Sy Bloom. I explained that I understood his decision and that I was determined to go home and work so hard that one day in the future he would have to name me to the team.

I told him that even at that time, Daphne didn't have to be constantly with me, but that I did need to have her help me with my bowel program.

Before I could say anything, he began to explain the decision.

"Skip, it's a very difficult decision that we made. I wish we could take you and some of the others. But we just don't have the facilities available for husbands and wives at this meet."

"Coach," I told him, "I understand your decision. I just came in to make sure you didn't think I had instigated what just happened.

"I'm going home to work as hard as I can, on my events and on taking care of myself, so that you'll have to select me one day. I have enough faith to believe that if I'm meant to be in the world games, I'll find a way to meet your needs."

Sy Bloom was pleasantly surprised and impressed.

"You've certainly got the right attitude. And you've got a lot of the right kind of faith. You're the kind of athlete we want on the U.S. team and I believe that you're going to get there one day.

"Thanks for understanding the decision."

21

We returned home in time for Shirley's graduation from Princess Anne. She had decided to go into nursing, which really pleased me, but didn't surprise me at all. She always had been the one who seemed eager to help me and she seemed more comfortable with some of the distasteful little things that I required.

Several days after Shirley's graduation, a letter from Sy arrived.

". . . there has been a cancellation by a competitor, we would like for you to be on the Paralympic team to compete in Toronto, Canada." He had remembered that I would need Daphne only sparingly for my personal needs.

Preparations for my first international trip required almost as much of my time indoors as outside on the practice field.

Wayne and I worked out every other day. We focused all of our attention on my form during the practice sessions. But we avoided going all-out, trying to throw for distance. That would come later when I was at the meet.

Daphne helped me try on and select the clothes I would need. Fashion had to yield to function. She sewed loops on my socks so I could get a finger through the loop and pull the socks up. She sewed large loops on the waist of my warmup pants, in the back. I could hook a finger in that loop to hike the pants up around my waist. I practiced over and over getting dressed and undressed. Whenever I ran into a problem, we improvised a solution.

Over and over I practiced each task that I would have to master to live alone. There were the pills. And the water jug. Handling the unexpected. The invitation to the games was forcing more and more independence on me.

It was rehearsal night for Skip. He was at home and Daphne was with him. But she was not to help him this night. He was on his own.

He pushed into the bathroom. He hooked his hands under his right leg and pulled it up, until his foot rested on a cross-brace of the chair. Using the life that had come back to his right hand from the operation, he reached down to the tube near his right ankle, unclamped it and drained his leg bag into the toilet.

He rinsed his hands and refilled his water jug at the sink. He would have to finish another half a gallon of water before bed to drink his daily intake of a gallon and a half.

Resting the jug in his lap, he rolled into the bedroom and pulled up to the nightstand. He reached in the drawer and pulled out a paper cup and the two rectangular plastic containers that held his pills. He opened a container. With his thumb and the first knuckle of his little finger on his right hand, he trapped a Vitamin C pill, raised it out of the container and dropped it into the paper cup. Now working with the back of his index finger, he isolated each kind of pill in the second container — Septa to ward off bladder infection, Vitamin E, Colace for softening his stool, and zinc to aid in healing anything that might be injured. One by one he dropped them into the paper cup. Then he emptied the contents of the cup in his mouth, swigged long on the jug and completed his nightly medical task. In another five minutes he had drained the contents of his third and final jug of water.

He maneuvered the transfer board into place on the bed — the mattress was high tonight. Other nights he had practiced with it being too low. Slowly he inched his body from his chair onto the bed.

He wormed and contorted himself out of his clothes, reached down for the blanket and pulled it completely over his body and head.

He had done it. The whole series of little duties and responsibilities that combined to make one full night of independent living.

He pulled the blanket back from his face. He and Daphne smiled at each other in triumph. But the sight of her so close to him, watching every move, acting as his safety net, made his smile fade. The next time he put himself to bed, she would be 30 miles away and he would be alone.

───────────

Despite my successful practice at home, waves of apprehension washed over me as I tried to imagine what kind of facilities awaited me. Daphne would be in the building with the coaches, administrators and family members of other athletes. Everything would have to be exactly right if I were to make it on my own.

My concentration on work at the Crisis Home and workouts with

Wayne was diverted shortly before I was to leave for Canada. Karen and Rob Ulsh were married in a large ceremony in Community Chapel and the days before the wedding were filled with family activity and happiness.

It wasn't until the day before I was to leave that I realized how much I would miss Wayne's companionship and help. He talked with me before I left.

"Skip, when your events start, you've got to forget everything that's going on around you. The biggest thing you have to remember is to concentrate. Concentrate on what you are doing. And what you are going to do. And really explode just at the end of each throw. And follow through. When you put it all together, from start to the follow through, that's when you get your best distances."

"I'll remember. I just wish you were going. Maybe one year you'll go into coaching," I said.

"Maybe. But I've got a long way to go. Nothing would be greater, though, than to be with you and Daphne."

The scene that unfolded when Daphne and I got our first view of the Olympic Village was staggering. I had never seen so many wheelchair athletes in one place. The registration procedure was exhausting. Both of us were already tired from travel; first to New York to assemble with the rest of the team, then on to Toronto. Two large circus tents had been set up for registration. We went from line to line, getting medical certification for my classification, having pictures taken, receiving room assignments. I had never been exposed to anything so large, so complex and so tiring.

My only thought was of rest. I had been sitting for 16 hours. I was beginning to worry about the callus. The roll from the registration area to the dorms seemed endless. I knew that Daphne was tired, too, but I didn't have the strength to wheel myself. Finally we arrived. I was in a small single room. She unpacked for me, located my clothes where I could reach them and kissed me goodbye. We didn't know when or where we would see each other again.

The aches in my body were soothed as soon as I was able to get myself onto the bed. The team meeting had lasted until after midnight. I was so exhausted that I almost decided to sleep in my clothes, but I forced myself to undress, to begin to live without help.

A knock on the door awakened me. Jack Whitman, one of the U.S. coaches and a former international competitor, wheeled inside to make sure that I had gotten through the night. After he left, I managed to dress and transfer myself into my chair. What I lacked in finesse I made up in determination. I was pleased and proud as I rolled to the door to begin the daily routine and workouts for my first international meet.

I wasn't accustomed to the demands of the practice sessions. We were up early, pushing long distances to the bus for the ride to the stadium, then sitting throughout the day as the teams worked out.

The hours of sitting in the chair took their toll. The callus on my rear split open. Before the competition started, I was worn out from the demanding daily routine, I saw Daphne infrequently, the callus was causing me physical and mental problems, and I had seen some of the best conditioned athletes in the world. My sole source of strength flowed from my reading of now-familiar Scriptures and frequent prayer.

I took special refuge in Paul's words in Second Corinthians, when he explains man's weakness in relation to Christ's strength:

> *"That is why, for Christ's sake, I delight in weaknesses, in insults, in hardships, in persecutions, in difficulties. For when I am weak, then I am strong."*

I received an emotional boost when I saw Mom and Dad on the opening day of competition. They had driven up from Virginia to be part of this event in my life. Becky and J.K. had come, too, all the way from Kentucky.

The boost wasn't enough, however. As the trials for the shot put began, I realized that the athletes gathered in Toronto were, indeed, the best in the world. Their form was more polished than mine, no matter what the cause of their disability. I was deflated at the end of the trials. I was in fourth place. Dad sensed that I was struggling. He came out of the stands and onto the field to encourage me. He reminded me that I was the best in the United States and that I could compete successfully with these athletes. But the tape measure told me otherwise. Just as I thought I had regained my composure, Weber, the German, smashed the existing world record in the shot. His throw traveled two feet further than the best throw I had ever made. I was still in fourth place after the finals ended. No medal.

I told myself that being fourth in the world was something to be proud of, but my emotions were deaf to that reasoning. My spirits sank even lower after the discus and club-throwing competition. I didn't reach the finals in either event.

Despite my poor showing, I was anxious to return home and start building myself. I had a much better understanding of what I needed to do to compete on the international level. I told Wayne about the athletes, their strength and their conditioning. I hoped that he could help me attain the kind of physical readiness I would need to succeed.

More than my renewed dedication to athletic excellence came out of the Toronto games. The opening and closing ceremonies were patterned after the pageanty that I had seen on television for the able-bodied Olympics. I was caught up in the majesty of the colors, the closing parade of athletes and the ceremony in which the Paralympic flame was extinguished. As I watched the American flag pass in review with the other countries and heard my National Anthem, I found it easy to be thankful for the days I had experienced.

"Lord," I prayed, "this is not the life I chose to live, but You have shown me that my life does have a purpose. I wouldn't miss this, even the pain of defeat, for anything."

I was close to tears. I realized that I felt so good about my life, even in a wheelchair, that I genuinely could be thankful to God. And even in a wheelchair, athletics was becoming a bigger and bigger part of my life.

I learned two lessons from my trip to Toronto.

The first lesson dealt with my physical abilities compared to my competitors. I knew that I had to develop more muscle and develop the ability to use that muscle. I changed my diet, eating balanced meals and shunning the sweets and pre-packaged snacks that had been frequent favorites.

I began to shed unneeded pounds. Wayne and I worked to transform fat into muscle. We obtained permission from my old high school,

Princess Anne, to use the weight room, and we set up a schedule of weight-training three days a week. Initially I started my workouts on a worn Universal Gym, using only 50 pounds in a seated military press. The first several days I had the same stiff and aching muscles that I had known in high school athletics. I enjoyed the soreness because I recognized the feeling; it was a soreness that came from physical training. The stiffness and the aching slowly disappeared and soon we added more weight to the lift, then added new exercises to the workouts. With each increment of weight that we added, we had proof that I was stronger. We made plans for a maximum of three regional meets for the upcoming season.

The second lesson that I learned from the Toronto trip was subtle; it required a lot of thought and reflection before it seeped into my mind. It dealt with spiritual growth.

Before I had gone to Canada, I had been meeting with Tom Rommelmeyer, a co-worker at the Crisis Home and a friend, in Bible study. I very much respected Tom's faith. His life was guided by daily prayer and his confidence in his relationship with God was something that I wanted to experience.

At the close of a study session together one afternoon, before I was to leave for the games, he said that he sensed, in his prayers for me, that my travel to Canada was not God's will. I was hurt and disappointed at what he told me, but I know that he had shared feelings only out of love and concern for me. I talked with others, whose faith had strengthened mine, about Tom's counsel. Their answers gave me no concrete guidance and didn't dispel my doubts about the trip and about my own faith. Why, I wondered, hadn't God spoken to *me* in some way about the trip? Was it that I didn't truly believe in Him? I had thought, until then, that I had matured in my understanding of God.

From the moment that I had arrived in Canada, I had been confused. My confidence about my faith was shaken. From the outset I had been plagued by disappointment. First the exhausting practices. Then the open sore. Finally, the defeats on the athletic field. Surely, from the evidence, my friend had been right.

I continued to think about the trip and its disappointments after I got home. Slowly, as I continued to study the Bible alone and with others, I began to see the trip and its events in a different light. Great benefits had come out of the trip. I had succeeded in taking care of myself without help. I had found strength in the words of the Bible when I was at a low point. I had tasted defeat in every event; yet my desire was to improve, not quit.

I began to understand that the trip had been a test for me.

Out of that test and the blessings I could now see in that trip, my faith in God grew in strength and in maturity. In the weeks that followed, I became excited because I knew that I was continuing to grow as a Christian. During these days of reflection and study, I committed myself to live my life to glorify God.

For many days after I made my commitment, I hoped for confirmation that my new athletic career was the way that I should glorify God. I wanted very much to remain in the world of competition. It had meant so much to me before the accident. It had given me something to strive for after I had begun to rebuild my body. Now, I felt, I was poised to make a real contribution in wheelchair sports.

The months of weight-training had given me strength. I now was pressing 100 pounds, twice the amount that I had started to work with. I was mentally and emotionally ready to face the kinds of exceptional competitors who had intimidated me in Canada.

There was no quick and convenient confirmation that athletics and my commitment to God were compatible. I returned over and over to the Scriptures and to prayer. I came to realize that, if I were to meet my commitment, I would have to put my faith in God, not in myself and my own acts. I finally understood how I would receive confirmation or denial from God about continuing my athletic work.

Wayne and I had decided on a minimum of two regional meets to gain experience. Three, perhaps, if we were doing well. The trips required considerable money; money that we did not have. In previous years, the funds had come to us in response to personal requests and as a result of newspaper articles about my efforts. I had met scores of people who had become supporters and friends and who were anxious to help me. I knew that I could call again on those who had helped in the past and that we would have the finances that we needed.

But I hesitated. Something inside me made me think about what I was doing and how I was going about it. I had reached the point in my life that I wanted to be certain that my efforts, no matter what they might be, were in keeping with God's purpose for my life.

I put the future of my athletics, actually all of my future, in God's hands.

I decided not to seek the needed funds from friends. I decided to take no initiative at all in raising the money. I believed that if it were God's will that I continue in athletics, He would somehow provide the means for me to compete. I believed just as strongly that if it were His will that I turn my life in another direction to serve Him, He would show me that new direction.

It was a big step for me to take, but my heart told me that I was ready to put all of my faith in God instead of myself, that I was ready to trust Him totally to know my needs and to help me meet them if He wanted me to pursue athletics in His name.

That decision took me to a new maturity in my Christian life. I not only could pray for such a sign, but I also could believe that He would show me a sign.

I realized that His answer to me could be an answer to end athletics. For a while I tried to anticipate how I would react if competition was not what God had in store. But I always returned to my willingness to accept whatever would glorify Him.

As far back as I could remember, I had never spent a prolonged time in worry about the difficulties I had experienced. There had been problems, to be sure. The frustrations in early athletics. The accident. The sickness that came with each bladder and kidney infection. The wound that at times split open from simply sitting in a wheelchair, bringing frustration and concern about athletics and my future health.

I now realized that each of these problems had its purpose for my life. They had led me, slowly and at times painfully, to a faith in God and to a desire to live my life for Him. I found reinforcement for my faith in the Bible. Often, during these weeks, I turned to a verse in Romans:

> *". . . all things work together for good to them that love God . . ."*

I also found reinforcement in my faith in weekly meetings with my friend Bud Hooper. Rob was completely involved in his youth work at Community Chapel and could no longer meet with us and Wayne's spiritual needs led him away from our meetings. Bud and I continued to talk about our lives as Christians. We talked about Scriptures and their meaning. We discussed books that had been written by others who had a faith.

I was at peace as Wayne and I continued to train. I didn't go to anyone for the money that we would need.

Wayne and I had moved our workouts out of doors as the weather warmed. With the winter of weight-training behind us, the next step was to put my new strength to work in the throwing circle. At the outset of our outdoor workouts, my throws were better than any of my past efforts, but there was no dramatic increase.

I was having lunch with Bob Dunsmore, the administrator for the Crisis Home system, one afternoon to review my programs. A local businessman, Aubrey Perry, stopped at the table. He was a Christian and had encouraged me in wheelchair sports. The three of us chatted for a few minutes, then Mr. Perry patted me on the shoulder and started to leave. He paused, then spoke to me.

"Skip, come by my office soon. I've got a check for you. For your traveling this year."

I was stunned.

"You do?" I knew the question sounded strange to him, but it was all that came out.

"Yes, I do." He smiled. "It will at least get you started."

I thanked him. As I spoke the words, I thanked God with all my heart. There was no question in my mind about the meaning of his gift. It was the first answer to my prayers. The first sign to appear.

Bob looked puzzled.

"Why the big smile? I've never seen you react exactly like that. You don't even know how much money he's donating for your trips."

"Bob, the amount doesn't matter," I said. "It could be five dollars, fifty dollars or five thousand dollars. I've just had a prayer answered and this is going to be a great year in wheelchair sports for me."

When I stopped by Mr. Perry's office several days later, I was given a check. A short note was attached to it. The note read, ''Good luck this year. God bless.'' The check was for $50.00

For an instant I was gripped by a doubt. Maybe God's true sign would be in the form of something dramatic, a fulfillment of all my financial needs at one time.

As I drove home, my mind turned over many of the lessons I had learned in the past years in Bible study. I focused again and again on a verse in Hebrews. Finally, it filled my mind and crowded everything else out:

> *''Faith is the substance of things hoped for, the evidence of things not seen.''*

I felt it was God's way of asking me, ''Don't you have enough faith to believe without evidence?'' I did. The doubt subsided. I truly didn't have much evidence to believe that it was God's will that I continue in athletics. When I completed my inventory that afternoon, I had listed $50.00 in cash and additional physical strength. I also listed a firm faith.

Four days later, after church, Bill Taylor came over to me. ''Skip, you've got to let me know when you need the money. I've got a list of people who want to help. They're just waiting to hear from me.''

I felt that God was speaking to me, saying, ''You see, have the faith to believe.''

The next day I telephoned Ran Randolph, the banker who had helped me with my travel funds in 1974. I asked him if the account was still active. He said that it was and he asked what I had in mind.

I told him only that I wanted to travel to several meets in the coming weeks and that some money had been donated for those trips. He was excited for me and told me that he would be happy to help in any way that he could.

A few minutes later, my phone rang. It was Ran. He asked for the details of my travel plans. I told him only where Wayne and I hoped to go.

''Skip, how are you going to raise that kind of money?''

I didn't answer his question; I was firm in my commitment not to seek help. Before I could say anything, he asked me to have lunch with him. He said he had an idea.

Ran and Jimmy Jordan, a marketing director with the bank, met me for lunch. I told them about some of my experiences in wheelchair sports and what I had learned about training since the last games. I shared with them my prayers for a Christian direction to my life.

Ran asked the question.

"Skip, have you ever spoken before a group of people before? About your experiences and the accident and your faith?"

"Yes, a couple of times."

"I think you ought to be speaking to a lot of people. They would appreciate knowing about your life; it's a great example of determination and faith. Plus the sports and what you have been able to do so far. I'd like to try to arrange for you to speak to some local groups, if you're interested."

After lunch, alone in my office, I thanked God for His answers to my prayer for a sign. I felt that He had shown me the direction that I should follow. He had led me to people who wanted to help. He had given me Ran Randolph and a way to raise funds.

Ran quickly went to work. He called the next day; he had talked with a member of the Virginia Beach Ruritan Club who wanted me to speak to that organization.

Ran, Wayne and I, accompanied by slides that Jimmy Jordan had taken of me in practice sessions, arrived on a Tuesday night for my talk.

Ran introduced me, telling the audience how he had come to know me. I prayed for God to give me the words to share with this group about me.

As I spoke, I sensed the attentiveness of the audience and I felt a confidence that I had never experienced before. It was a good feeling, a feeling that I was doing what I should be doing. I told my story and gave them a glimpse of wheelchair athletics. I told them that I felt I could be a champion one day. It wasn't a boast. It just came out as a quiet statement. I hadn't planned to say it.

After my talk, I answered a lot of questions about my personal and athletic life.

Ran closed their program by telling the club of my financial needs for travel. Before we left, Ran received a donation from the club for

$250.00. Many individual members told him that they wanted to contribute, too.

Ran called me at home that night to tell me how well he thought I had spoken. He was convinced that he could help me raise all of the money that would be required if I would share with others as I had shared with the Ruritan Club. Just saying "Thank You" to Ran seemed a small way to tell him how much I appreciated his help, but I think he understood.

One speaking engagement led to another. The newspapers picked up my story and local television stations asked me to appear and share my story with their audiences. It was an exciting time. Soon I had received enough contributions to insure travel to our first regional meet. I also received something far more important than the funds. I received acknowledgement that the way I was trying to live my life was worthwhile to others. Most of the people who contributed knew very little about wheelchair sports. By the notes they wrote to me and the words they said, I knew that they were interested in me and what I was doing with my life.

Part Four

22

I had the first shift behind the wheel of the van as Wayne, Daphne and I left Virginia Beach late Thursday night, April 25, 1977, to drive to the season's first regional meet at Ohio State University in Columbus.

Daphne had already stretched out in the back of the van to sleep before her turn behind the wheel came. I had cleared most of the city traffic coming out of Norfolk before Wayne broke the silence.

"Skip," he said, "you're going to break some records at this meet. I can sense it."

I thought for a minute before I answered.

"This *is* the big test. If I can put it all together, I might. We've come a long way. I think maybe I *can* break some records."

I had a new confidence about my ability and about what I was doing in athletics. Wayne and I had developed a more powerful throwing technique for my field events. My question to God about the rightness of my competition had brought back His answer in the form of travel funds and encouragement.

As I drove toward our first stop, Kentucky, and an overnight stay with Becky and J.K. Pell, Wayne and I reminisced about a Sunday afternoon, only four weeks before in Bud Hooper's backyard.

The day was unusually warm for March, but a strong wind was blowing. Bud's yard was sheltered by neighboring houses and trees. It wasn't large enough for me to throw the club, but I had plenty of room to practice the shot and the javelin and discus.

We had been practicing for more than two hours and we were tired. We also were frustrated. I was a lot stronger. I could feel it every time I threw. But the new strength hadn't improved my performance very much in any of the events.

Wayne was sitting at the foot of my chair; the equipment was spread out in front of me on the ground.

"Something's missing, Skip. Maybe I'm overlooking something." Wayne said, looking at the ground and idly pulling at blades of grass.

"I don't know. Maybe it's in my form? You know, I noticed that a lot of the athletes, some with less disability than me, sit farther forward in their chairs than I do. They angle their chairs in the circle so they're throwing almost over the back of their chairs.''

Wayne stopped pulling at the grass and looked up. ''Say that again.''

''I'll show you. Here, get up and turn my chair.''

We angled the chair so that I faced almost 180 degrees away from the throwing area. I inched my body to the front of the chair.

I moved slowly through the motions of putting the shot. The new position was awkward. I had always had the left side of the chair perpendicular to the throwing area. I noticed something else, too. Even though I was putting very little pressure against the chair, the chair tipped.

''Wayne, I can't throw anything unless you hold the chair.'' I went through the throwing motion again and Wayne quickly saw what I meant.

''Okay, I see what you mean. Here. Let's try one and see what happens.'' He handed me the shot and sat on the ground, grabbing the chair with both hands and bracing it with his feet.

I threw. The shot went higher than usual, but it didn't appear to travel any farther.

I tried again. Again the shot went higher, but apparently no farther.

''Let's mark three just to see if there's any difference,'' Wayne said.

I put everything into the three throws. I pinned the end of the tape at the base of the chair with the javelin. Wayne reeled out the tape and walked to the spot where the first and closest shot had landed. In practice sessions, he kept the tape about waist-high, eyeballed the distance and yelled it back to me. This time he eyeballed it, then kneeled down and put the tape to the ground, getting an exact measurement. He looked back with a puzzled expression, then moved to the second spot. When he looked up again, his puzzlement had been replaced by a slight smile.

He stood up after the third measurement.

''This one is over 16 feet. They're all better than anything you've ever thrown.''

''You're kidding!'' But I knew that he wouldn't kid about something that serious.

We wanted to get excited, but we couldn't believe that such an adjustment in chair position would make such a difference.

I hurried through three more throws. The results were the same. Two of the throws were close to 16 feet; the third was just over the 16-foot mark.

We stopped for a minute to rest and to relish what had just happened. We had the same questions on our minds: Was it chance? A fluke? Had we measured right? Could I do it again?

We moved to the discus, then the javelin. Each time I went to a new event, at least one of my efforts in the backyard of the Hooper residence broke a national record.

A bruise was developing on my chest where it hit the back of the chair at the end of each throw, but I kept going. We worked until dark.

We practiced the next day at lunch outside the Crisis Home. We were still afraid that we would lose whatever we had found. But the shot throws again were near or over the 16-foot mark.

"We've got it. We've got it, Wayne. This is the breakthrough. I can do it. I can do it consistently. We're not going to lose it," I said.

We didn't lose it. Each practice confirmed that we had reached a new plateau. There was always a feeling of relief, though, when the tape measure confirmed that I had, indeed, improved.

A steady cold rain fell in Columbus as we waited in the van, watching the events on the field in front of us. I was nervous. I kept pushing out of my mind the thought that maybe the rain or the cold would make a difference, that perhaps I could only hold my improved form in warm, dry weather.

My first event was the javelin. At the end of my three throws, I had broken the national record of 32 feet, 10 inches. My throw was 33 feet, 9 inches.

The shot put was next. I threw 16 feet, breaking the national record of 14 feet, 5 inches that I had set.

I didn't set a national record in the discus, but I won the event with a throw of 31 feet, 2 inches.

I won the club throw and the precision club throw.

The next day I won the table tennis singles.

At the banquet that night I learned that my six gold medals had put my individual performance in third place in *team* competition.

Fishersville was next and Mom and Dad were in the crowd of spectators.

I bettered my Ohio performances. I broke national records in the shot with a throw of 16 feet, 11½ inches; the javelin with 34 feet, 3 inches; the discus with a throw of 36 feet, 2 inches; and the club with a throw of 65 feet, 1 inch. I won the table tennis singles.

Wayne and I decided to go to a third regional, the one in New York. It would be an opportunity to gain more experience with the new form and improve my chances — if I did well — of being selected for the U.S. team.

I was speaking two and three times a week to local groups, thanks to Ran's interest in me. I realized that people were expressing interest in my story for more than just the medals and records that were beginning to come to me. More and more, I lived my life for God. I never worked out or competed that I didn't say a quiet prayer from Scriptures to remind myself of His blessings: "And whatsoever ye do, do it heartily, as to the Lord, and not unto men . . ."

I was finding joy in living a Christian life.

The New York trip was going to be expensive and I was careful about how I spent the funds that had been donated. Another prayer was answered when I called Steve Kemp. I had met him at the 1976 Paralympics in Canada. He was a New York fireman and had been injured when he fell through a roof fighting a house fire. He had planned to compete at Long Island, but had been blessed by muscle return in much of his body. His injury had turned out to be a temporary one and he was recovering so rapidly that he would no longer compete in wheelchair athletics. His former sponsor offered to defray some of my travel expenses to Long Island.

As my faith had grown, my view of wheelchair sports had changed. I looked on the opportunity to compete as an opportunity for anyone who was disabled to rebuild confidence in himself, as well as rebuild his body. I was proud to be part of the effort and I had pride for everyone who participated. It didn't matter to me how well someone did as long as he tried. We applauded each other's efforts, receiving and giving strength to each other. At Eisenhower State Park on Long Island, I learned how important such an attitude could be to others in wheelchairs.

Wayne and I were studying the shot-putters at Eisenhower as I waited for my name to be called. Some of them had to struggle to heave the shot a few precious feet from their chairs. There was an athlete sitting near me. I had seen him warming up and he was unusually strong and agile for the 1Λ classification. Each time a throw went only a short distance, he made a disparaging remark. I could tell that his comments hurt some of the competitors.

His turn in the circle came before mine and his first throw was a good one. He turned to the crowd of athletes as if to boast, "How'd you like that one?" He was good. But my heart ached for the others whom he had ridiculed. If I had needed any extra incentive, he provided it.

Wayne leaned over to me when my name was called to enter the circle.

"We've got to shut that guy up, Skip. What a jerk."

I knew that my first throw was going to be a record when the shot left my hand. My body had functioned perfectly and every ounce of strength went into the throw. The official had hardly called out the distance — "18 feet, 1½ inches" — when I heard behind me, "That guy's no 1A. He's in the wrong classification." I knew who had shouted the remark. It didn't bother me; the other athletes wheeled up to congratulate me.

My throw had been farther than the world record and I had unofficially set a new world mark. I broke national records in the shot, club and javelin and I set a regional record in the discus. I won the table tennis competition later that night.

Wayne and I had planned to return to Virginia Beach the next morning, but meet officials asked us to stay until the end of all of the competition. The reason for their request became apparent at the end of the meet. I was awarded the Alonzo Wilkins Award, given to the meet's outstanding athlete based on performance, character and sportsmanship.

As important as the award to my increasing confidence about athletic competition, there was something more important that was given to me before Wayne and I left for the long trip home.

As I held the award in my hands, the athletes who had been the objects of earlier scorn and ridicule by one of us came over to me. They wanted me to know that they appreciated the fact that I had come all the way to Long Island and that I really deserved the award.

23

Soon after I returned from the New York meet, Wayne and I and three wheelchair athletes from the Beach — Don Davidson, Roger Payne and Ronnie Kirkland — got together to form a local wheelchair team. The four of us had competed in some of the same meets in the past, but we had entered as individuals. Wayne offered to help the other three with training and coaching. The five of us became the founding members of the Virginia Beach Sun Wheelers.

We went to the nationals in San Jose as a team. Everything seemed to be working for me, and there was the thrill of a very personal competition to add to the excitement of the nationals. Fred McBee, an athlete from Tampa, Florida, and I had become friendly competitors during the 1976 national games. Before we left the nationals, Fred had issued a friendly challenge: he was going to beat me in the shot the next time we met. That meeting came in San Jose.

I took first in the shot, breaking the record, and Fred came in right behind me. It was the same in the javelin. I broke the record and Fred was second. The club throw was the final event of the meet for our 1A class. It was a dramatic example of the best kind of competition. Fred had made his last throw in the finals and had broken the record with a toss of 64 feet, 5 inches. On my third and last throw in the finals, I hit a mark of 65 feet, 10 inches, beating Fred and breaking the record he had set.

Both of us had wanted the gold medal and we had pushed ourselves as hard as we could. When it was over, we were still friends and we were pleased for each other's performances. Fred reminded me, with a smile, that I had a lot of work to do in table tennis before I could defeat him. He had beaten me in that event the day before to take a gold medal.

I tried to relax as Daphne and I sat at the table, waiting for the awards banquet to begin the final night in San Jose. I was at peace with myself about my performances. I had done as well as I could and I felt that the three new records I had set were added tributes to share with my family and with God. I wanted very much to go to the World Games, but word was already out that the U.S. team would be one of the smallest in history; no more than 25 athletes.

I was talking with Daphne about the next day's flight to Colorado when I felt a hand on my shoulder. I looked up and into the smiling face of Sy Bloom. He had stopped on his way to the head table.

He leaned down close to my ear and whispered.

''Skip, can you go to England this year?''

His smile grew, he patted me on the shoulder and disappeared toward his table. He had left me with the advance knowledge that I would be a member of the 1977 U.S. wheelchair team before he announced the names to the audience.

The callus on my rear had split again during the competition. I hadn't let it affect my attitude during the games, but I wouldn't accept the fact that I would have to worry about it splitting open every time I competed. There had to be a solution. One of the door prizes at the final banquet was a Roho cushion. I had heard of them and when I examined it, I thought it might be the answer to my problem. I didn't win the door prize, but I left California determined to get one and try a cushion. We landed in Denver to visit Daphne's sister and brother-in-law, Debbie and Michael Tanner, in Greeley, Colorado. I called Roho headquarters in St. Louis, Missouri. Otto Roberts, the vice president, came on the phone to talk to me. He had read about me in Sports 'N' Spokes, a bimonthly magazine about wheelchair athletes, and he said that he would send a cushion to my home in Virginia Beach. When we arrived, the cushion was there. After I had used it a short time, I knew that it was the solution to an old and nagging problem.

I preceded Daphne and Wayne to England, making my first trip alone. The first few days, trying to take care of all of my personal needs without Daphne's help, were vivid reminders of how very much she meant to me and how many things she did to insure my comfort.

Wayne used his own money and came as a guest. He was working hard to become a recognized coach to me. He spent his spare time talking to other coaches and to athletes and studying the forms of the better athletes.

I was defeated in the first round in singles table tennis and managed only a fourth place in the discus and club. There was no javelin throw in the world games. I won my first world medal in the shot, coming in second behind Weber, the German. And Rod Vleiger and I won the gold in team table tennis, the first time I had competed in the event.

It was a rewarding meet. My marks had been consistent with my performances in the regionals. More importantly, I didn't have any trouble with the callus.

The world games ended the year's competitions. My weekend training sessions were replaced by lazy weekends at Carolina, fishing with Wayne and Mike Preziotti.

Daphne and I daily gave thanks for the blessings that we now had. My accident, the operations, the pain, and the fear of death all seemed so far in the past. I did not expect any greater happiness than we had. But more was to come.

The phone rang one evening and a man introduced himself to me as Pete Marx. He said that he had followed my high school athletic career and had followed my efforts in wheelchair sports. He made an appointment to have lunch with me.

When I met Pete Marx, I instantly liked him. He was motivated by the joy of helping others. He wanted to do something for me. He asked about my background, about the accident and how I had worked to overcome my handicaps. He wanted the Norfolk Sports Club to honor me in some way, perhaps with a special Skip Wilkins Day. I was flattered at his thoughtfulness. His interest made me realize again how much I had to be thankful for, but I didn't dwell on the possible honor.

Weeks later the phone rang as Daphne and I were finishing dinner. The caller introduced himself as Rob Barton of the Virginia Beach Jaycees.

"Skip," he said, "on behalf of the Jaycees, I'd like to invite you to be our guest at a banquet on November 22nd . . ."

I interrupted him to ask Daphne for a pen and paper. When I told her that it was the Jaycees, a look of anticipation came over her.

Rob repeated the details of time, date and place.

"Skip, what I am about to tell you is in confidence. We haven't said anything to the papers yet."

I didn't understand what he had said or why, but I did hear and understand the next sentence.

"Skip, you have been chosen the Outstanding Young Man of Virginia Beach."

I couldn't speak. I was overwhelmed. I looked at Daphne. Tears streamed down her face. She had known what the call was about.

My shock gave way to joy. I had a hard time concentrating on the rest of the conversation, but I remembered clearly the names of the two people Rob said had nominated me: Bill Taylor and Pete Marx.

The Jaycees banquet was like a family reunion. Linda and Tommy, Karen and Rob, Shirley, Granny and Papa, Mom and Dad, and Daphne and I were at one table. The room was crowded and everywhere I glanced I saw someone who had helped me, who had encouraged me on the journey back from the bottom of the lake.

The speaking engagements that Ran had arranged earlier in the year had helped me become increasingly comfortable as a speaker. I sensed that I had a worthwhile message to share when I spoke. People wanted to hear me. I never wrote out any speeches or made notes. I asked myself one question before I spoke: what do I want to share? I would pray for God to provide the right word for my message.

I had known what I wanted to share at the Jaycees' banquet as soon as I had recovered from the shock of Rob Barton's phone call.

As I was introduced, I silently thanked God once again for giving me the opportunity to speak the words I was about to speak. So much had happened to me, so much had been done for me. Now, on this night so close to Thanksgiving, I could give thanks in public to my family for their love and their care.

Skip rolled to a stop in front of the podium and took the microphone that was handed to him.

He looked out across the audience, still standing and applauding at their places at the tables.

"I am very honored to receive this award tonight. In accepting it, I would like to honor those who have made my life possible, because these people are what is truly outstanding about my life."

He turned to the table where his family sat and looked at his parents.

"I was fortunate to have parents who did not panic at the time of the accident. When my life suddenly came to a halt and death was so close, they gave me hope. I am thankful to them for they made me feel accepted as I struggled to accept myself."

He looked at Shirley, Karen and Linda.

"I am thankful for my three sisters, who had to give up many of their wants and needs and assume the responsibilities of caring for each other and the home. When I came home, they were the ones to care for me and help me. Linda, my oldest sister, drove me to college every morning before going to school herself."

He turned to his grandparents.

"My grandparents gave of themselves, too. They taught me a great lesson in giving as they sacrificed to give me money and support to carry on a normal life."

Skip's eyes focused on Daphne.

"My wife has been always supportive and encouraging. What has been accomplished, we have accomplished together. She is truly the person who makes me complete.

"It is because of this love and the pulling together and the working together that I have been able to make something out of my life."

Skip looked again across the audience.

"There, of course, have been others who have helped me tremendously, but to try to name them all would be difficult.

"Just today, I tried to write a person who has helped me over the past few months."

Skip's gaze came to rest for a moment on Ran Randolph.

"This person has become a true friend, but I could not find the proper words to say on paper. But again, it is because of people caring for me that I have been allowed to achieve the things that I have.

"So, tonight, I would like to thank the Virginia Beach Jaycees for the honor of Outstanding Young Man of Virginia Beach because, by honoring me, you are really giving the honor to my family and my friends."

24

The first recognition solely for my athletic efforts came in January 1978. The Norfolk Sports Club designated a Skip Wilkins Day. Pete Marx again was responsible for the tribute. George McClelland, the sports editor of *The Virginian-Pilot,* attended. The next morning he wrote in his column:

> Not long ago Skip Wilkins helped his alma mater, Princess Anne High School, form a Fellowship of Christian Athletes chapter.
>
> He undertook the project, he confesses, with some misgivings.
>
> "I thought," confides this young man who has turned his wheelchair from a prison into a chariot dedicated to the Lord's work, "that we might draw a handful of puny kids. Instead, we had about 50 of the top athletes in school.
>
> "Now we have a vigorous chapter there, and four other schools in Virginia Beach have asked me to help them with similar programs."
>
> If Alfred Thomas Wilkins' voice is edged in wonder, it is because this young man with the message of hope and faith underestimates the ease with which he ferrets out man's nobler instincts.
>
> This was Monday at the Norfolk Sports Club . . .
>
> The return to athletics came four years ago. By 1974 he was ready to enter the first Virginia Regional Wheelchair Games. In another year he was qualified for national competition. Coached by Wayne Whitley and encouraged by his wife and family, Wilkins has progressed to a point that he is one of the foremost quadriplegic athletes in the country. Tomorrow the world.

But the roses have a different, a sweeter, smell.
"It's really neat to compete against people
I can help.
"I hope handicapped people come to real-
ize that other people care and are concerned.
"Trying is what it's all about.
"Touching lives, too.
"I don't know what the future holds, but
I'm excited about it."
Skip Wilkins is forced neither to reach nor
to stoop to conquer. He has rolled over fear
and despair and frustration. He will dispose of
similar obstacles without flinching.

I had received enormous courtesy and coverage from the two Norfolk newspapers, but George's words had a special meaning to me
because they spoke of me as an athlete who wanted to help others.

Several weeks later I was surprised at the Virginia Beach Sports
Club's annual Jamboree. Daphne and I attended because the club had
made me an honorary member the year before, after I had spoken to the
members. Mom and Dad attended the banquet, too, which was a bit
unusual. Bill McDaniel began the introduction of the Sportsman of the
Year.

"Next year, when the description of tonight's 1978 Sportsman of
the Year is printed in our program, we are going to add the words
'motivation' and 'inspiration' because that's what this young man is all
about."

He turned in my direction.

It was only then that I realized that I was being honored. Daphne,
Mom and Dad had known about the honor for days, but they were as
touched as I was when it was announced.

Weeks later, Ran Randolph was waiting outside my office at the
Crisis Home on a cold, rainy day in February. I had been director of the
home for almost three years. I had a staff of seven counselors. They
cared for and provided counseling help, around the clock, for as many
as 15 children at one time.

We had been successful in returning many youngsters to their homes, after helping them to calm down from an immediate crisis and to understand how to deal with future problems. Some of them couldn't adjust; others refused to help themselves. These had to be returned to the courts for further consideration. I had become accustomed to their often explosive tempers, even violence at times, but I had deep regrets when we had to return a child to the court.

I had just finished a difficult conversation with a youngster who was headed back to court for his constant aggressive behavior toward other children.

Ran was about to come into the office when a staff member stormed in, quickly became belligerent and proceeded to complain about the salary that she was paid. She was hostile and abusive. My stern reminder to her that she had been aware of the salary when she had sought the position finally dampened her anger and she finally returned to her duties.

On the way to lunch, Ran turned to me.

"Skip, I don't see how you do it. Putting up with that kind of abuse day in, day out. You know, you have so much more to offer."

I didn't understand.

He explained what was on his mind.

"I've heard a lot of inspirational speakers, Skip. But I am moved each time I hear you tell your story. And I've heard you speak now . . . what, about 30 times? With the gift that you have, I mean speaking, perhaps a book, you could have anything you want."

I thought for a minute.

"Ran, it's not the material things. A million dollars or anything else that you can name wouldn't let me walk again. What's important is what I do with what I have. I'm happy now and I have a contentment I have never known before."

"How," he asked, "can you have such a peace after what you've been through?"

"I didn't always have it, you know that. It only came when I realized that something was missing and I asked God to forgive me and to direct my life. It isn't always easy, but I feel that I'm living for Him."

"I wish I had that kind of peace. There're so many things that I worry about," he said.

"I can't give it to you. You have to ask for it for yourself. But I can help you learn about it. All you have to do is make a commitment of time to learn with me what the Bible says about it."

Ran agreed and our lunch ended on a happy and thoughtful note. I was glad that I could be of some help to Ran as we discussed a schedule for Bible study.

Later, back in my office, I thought about Ran's comments on my speaking. I genuinely enjoyed sharing my story and the joy of my faith with others. During the past year my belief had grown stronger and stronger that God had given me a special gift in the story of my life, that it was His will that I meet with others and share His blessings on me and my family.

Word of my speaking continued to spread, even beyond the community and the state, and the requests to speak increased. Ran, at lunch on that rainy day that had started with problems at the Crisis Home, had helped me focus on the possibility of a broader ministry for God.

My spring weight-training and the workouts with Wayne paid off in a big way when 1978 competition began. Wayne had left the Crisis Home and had become a full-time therapeutics specialist with the Parks and Recreation Department of Virginia Beach. He worked exclusively in wheelchair sports.

I won six gold medals in the regionals at Long Island. The shot, discus, club and singles table tennis continued to be my best events. The javelin had been dropped as an event, but I competed in two races, the 60-yard dash and the 220-yard dash, and managed two firsts in those events.

I repeated with six victories at the regionals at Fishersville and Clearfield, Pennsylvania.

Tommy Wilkins had propped his back against the side of the van, his legs stretched on the floor in front of him. Skip was lying on the back seat next to him.

The trip to Clearfield had erased weariness and worry from Tommy.

He'd been able to relax, even to laugh at some of the antics that had been part of the stay with Skip, Wayne and Ed Sadler.

Skip had done so well. Six gold medals. He looked over at his son who was awake.

Tommy wanted to talk. He'd kept so much to himself until now.

"You know, Skip, I think I'm just now getting over what we've been through. The whole family. I've never talked much about the accident, but it might help if I shared some of the things that I've tried to deal with."

He didn't wait for a response.

"I didn't have much of a life when I was young. No father when I really needed one. I guess I felt I had to do everything for myself. I had to prove that I was a man. That's one reason I was so stern with you when you were growing up. I wanted you to know about discipline and rules. That's part of life.

"And there's another big thing, too. You may already understand it because of what we've been through. You were my son. You were an extension of my life. You were the one person I cared more about than anyone else. Your life and your athletics were everything to me. You were doing what I wished I had done when I was young.

"The accident took all of that away from me. All I had left for a while was a lot of pain and a lot of questions. But you know, I never questioned God. Not once. I used to go to the chapel in Norfolk General every time I came to see you. Nobody knows that. I didn't want them to. I'm not sure why.

"It was pretty lonely, too. I had a lot of decisions to make. And I didn't know much about what had happened to you. I mean medically. How things would turn out. A lot of the time I felt that the whole thing was on me. That nobody but me could help you. But I felt so helpless myself. It took a lot out of me. A lot more than I realized, I guess.

"But you've come back now. You'll never know what a thrill it was to watch you in the meet. I never thought we'd have these kinds of times again.

"But the most important thing I want to tell you is about the family. We need to work together to take care of the family. You never know when something might happen. Just like your accident. We've got to always be thinking what we're going to do for the family today. All of us are so important to each other.''

Skip looked at his dad and nodded that he understood what he had heard. That was all that he could do.

The accident had touched so many lives and brought so many feelings to the surface. Pain. Anger. Frustration. Compassion. Love. Humor.

''Yes, even some humor,'' Skip thought.

There was the Case of the Broken Bone. That had been in 1969 when Skip had tumbled from his wheelchair on a gambol with classmates through the state park. That night his right leg began jumping into the air, sometimes as high as a foot. Everybody got excited. Was Skip getting return? The leg had to be tied to the chair for the next day's classes. An afternoon visit to the doctor explained the reason. Skip had fractured his foot in his tumble. He couldn't feel the pain, of course. That was it: no return, which nobody really had expected, but the awareness that a broken foot would never hurt.

Then there was the Episode of the Stuffed Sock. His leg started a similar action in class a couple of years later. He knew that he hadn't broken any bones this time. Maybe this time he was getting some return. What else could it be? The answer came when Skip was preparing for bed. What it turned out to be, was a sock. A brown sock. In the hurry of dressing him that morning, Patsy had left a sock stuffed in the toe of a shoe. The pressure and the cramping through the day had brought about the reaction in the leg.

In 1976 there had been the False Alarm Caper. Linda had brought her 2-year-old daughter, Kari, to visit. Kari had gone into Skip's room early in the morning to peep at her uncle, still asleep. When she left she closed the door. It locked.

Patsy discovered the locked door when she went to awaken Skip.

''Skippy, you remember how we've talked about what you would do if you were alone and the house caught on fire?'' she called, loud enough to wake him up.

''Yeah, Mom. Why?''

Patsy, Linda and Kari, who quickly began to mimick her mother and grandmother, stood outside the door, yelling. ''Fire! Fire!''

Skip's chair had been left at the dresser. He snared it with a long dowel rod with a saucer hook on the end and pulled it to the bedside. It took him several minutes to transfer and roll to the door.

When he opened it, there was no fire. Only laughter.

"I didn't know what else to do," Patsy said. "And I thought you'd probably stay in bed all day if I told you that I couldn't get in."

After the laughter died away, they resolved that the chair would always be left beside his bed and that the lock on the door would be made inoperative.

Perhaps the funniest, at least to Skip, was the Case of Mistaken Identity in 1971.

Skip had gone to DePaul Hospital to visit a friend. As he rolled down the hall on the pediatric floor looking for the room, a nurse had passed him.

"Young man, you'll have to get out of that chair. They're reserved for patients."

He didn't have time to explain before she continued on her way.

Several minutes later, the nurse reappeared. She had another nurse with her. A large woman. Very stern.

"Young man, I'll have to insist that you get out of that chair right now. They're not for visitors to play with. They're for the patients who need them."

Skip looked at the two women and started to laugh.

"Nurse," Skip said, "I've been trying to get out of this thing for the past four years."

The nationals were held at Fishersville in June. I won a gold in the shot, the club and singles table tennis and was selected for the U.S. team that would compete in the 1978 Pan American games in Rio de Janeiro.

It was in Fishersville at the nationals that I received reinforcement that I could touch people and that my message, with God's help, could be a message of hope to others.

I had appeared on a Christian television program, The 700 Club hosted by Pat Robertson, in April 1978 and had told the story of my accident and the decision to give my life to the Lord.

Several of the athletes who competed at Fishersville came to me during the meet and told me that they, too, were Christians and that they had received encouragement and support when they had heard me on the program. The bonds that had tied us together, our wheelchairs and our athletics, became much stronger because of a spiritual understanding.

Daphne and I went to Elizabethtown, Pennsylvania, before our trip to Brazil. The Fellowship of Christian Athletes had asked us to speak to their first summer conference for girls. I had worked since 1974 on behalf of the FCA's high school organizations. Through my association with the Fellowship, I had been enriched with the friendships of Christians who were athletes at all levels. It was Daphne's first appearance before a large group. After I had shared the story of my life with the conference, she related the story of her acceptance of God and told them something about the life of an athlete's wife. We received a standing ovation at the end of her talk, but I doubt that anyone was more appreciative of her talk than I was. It was a beautiful time for us, being with old and new friends and being able to tell of the wonderful things that were happening to us as husband and wife.

The flight to Rio with Daphne was especially enjoyable because we were leaving the United States for the first time as a couple, but I found myself in the middle of chaos and confusion shortly after we landed. The U.S. team was assigned to the second floor of a barracks building far from downtown Rio. There were no elevators and each of us had to negotiate a series of sharp turns to get up a steep two-story ramp outside the building. I was exhausted from the trip and the sweltering heat. Once inside I realized that any rest would be a long time in coming. The whole team was in one large room with bunk beds. The bottom beds were too low and the top bunks were too high for easy transfer.

Wayne had been selected as a U.S. coach for the Pan American games and I was thankful that he was with me. I managed, under his watchful eye, to maneuver into a lower bunk. I had hardly put my head on the pillow to rest when the bunk collapsed to the floor. Shortly after this accident, other beds began breaking as athletes sought relief from the weariness of travel and the heat. An official of the host country appeared and advised us that the plumbing was not in the best working order. We had already been advised to drink only bottled water. All of us were accustomed to hardships, but in quick succession we had been confronted with a ramp as steep as a mountain, beds that were turning into splinters, no working toilets, warnings against the drinking water and armed guards standing watch over the barracks.

Athletes began to protest the conditions; some threatened to go home. Wayne and I moved off to a corner of the dormitory and I was able to lie down and begin to rest. As tired as I was, my mind flashed back to a conversation that I had with Bud Hooper shortly before I left the States.

He had recommended some Scriptures to me. I turned to the first chapter of Colossians and began reading the ninth verse. The words, as Bud had told me, brought a sense of peace and strength amid the confusion and growing discontent in the dormitory:

> *". . . in order that you may live a life worthy of the Lord and may please Him in every way: bearing fruit in every good work, growing in the knowledge of God, being strengthened with all power according to His glorious might so that you may have great endurance and patience . . ."*

As soon as Ben Lipton, administrator of the U.S. team, learned of the conditions that surrounded the team, he called us together.

"We have two options," he told the assembled athletes. "We can either stay here and make the best of it . . . or we can try to find accommodations in a motel. If we move to a motel, we'll have to go home and get contributions to cover the additional money that it's going to cost. We just don't have the money to pay for those kinds of rooms. I'll have to have a unanimous vote from the team, no matter what is decided."

When Ben called for the first vote, the one to move to a different location, every hand shot into the air. We couldn't move out fast enough. We were relocated in a motel in Rio and I was able to stay with Daphne. The motel offered a beautiful view of the ocean and the food was plentiful and excellent.

While we won a victory over the poor housing, none of us from

America sucessfully combatted the heat. It was constant and drained our strength. We soaked our T-shirts in water. Minutes later, they were bone dry. The athletes especially sensitive to hot temperatures constantly sought whatever slight shade or breeze available. I spent most of my time between events waiting under a section of the bleachers where there was often a slight breeze.

The outdoor thermometer reached 104 degrees on the morning of the shot put. I felt my strength being sapped by the heat as I waited for my turn. There was no breeze. A single small cloud drifted across the sun as I made my throws. The sudden relief from the blazing sun brought me physical and psychological relief. I won the gold, breaking the Pan American record with a throw of 5.50 meters.

At the end of the meet, I had won another gold in the 4 by 60-meter relay, a silver in the discus and the team table tennis, and a bronze in the 60-meter race and the singles table tennis.

When Daphne and I returned to Virginia Beach, it was to a far different place than the dormitory room in Rio. Dad had built a ground-level duplex apartment next to the house. One side had received new tenants in October: Mr. and Mrs. Alfred T. Wilkins Jr. Daphne and I had truly returned to our home.

25

I was invited to return to the Norfolk Sports Club in late January 1979 as one of a number of local and national celebrities. We had gathered to help the club celebrate its annual day-long sports Jamboree, one of the largest in the nation. During the morning session and again at the luncheon, I was aware that a great deal of attention was being paid to me by local media. I was puzzled by it, but as the afternoon progressed, I gave it no more thought.

That night, at the Jamboree banquet, I discovered why so many reporters had chatted with me and why so many photographers had asked me to pose with some of the national athletes in attendance. I received another unexpected honor. Rawlings Keefe, at the head table, had not finished his introductory remarks of the club's Sportsman of the Year when I realized, from his description, that the club was honoring me. Dad was seated in a far corner of the banquet room. Wayne had been unable to attend. This latest tribute gave me the opportunity publicly to thank Wayne, even though he couldn't be there to hear me, for his encouragement and his help in my athletic career and to honor Dad once again for his love and his determination.

I remember saying, as I looked at Dad in the far corner of the crowded room, "I am thankful to my Dad. He gave me the encouragement and the help to go on when it would have been so easy to give up." No matter how many opportunities came to me to tell others about my family's love and devotion, I knew that I would always sense a welling up of love and pride each time I told of their sacrifices. That feeling of love for them became one more reason I wanted to share my life and give encouragement and inspiration to others.

The desire to build a speaking career came a step closer to reality in February 1979. I sensed that my time at the Crisis Home was nearing an end. For four years I had worked to build the staff and to improve the facilities and the program. I felt that I had successfully met the challenges that had faced me as the home's founding director. I continued to be rewarded by the daily efforts to help the young people in our care. Each time a child showed improved behavior, each time a youngster began to open his feelings to the staff and show improvement, all of us shared a sense of accomplishment.

But the responsibility of shaping the home and giving it direction had largely been met. I felt that I should concentrate my goals on helping others by speaking and sharing the joys that I had found in living my life.

Ran again was instrumental in bringing me to a big decision. He asked me to meet with Jimmy Jordan again. Jimmy had left the bank to put together, with his brother Fred, a small publishing firm in Virginia Beach. When he heard that I was considering leaving the Crisis Home, he asked me to consider joining the new company. He wanted me to think about sharing the story of my life in a book and he was excited about my growing interest in meeting and speaking with groups and individuals. In addition, he wanted to make time available to me to continue to compete in wheelchair games, as long as I felt there was a purpose beyond the awards. The offer seemed like an answer to my prayers about how best to use my life. I discussed the opportunity with Daphne and Dad. They, like me, thought it would be the right thing to do. I joined the firm in April and soon began to work on organizing my thoughts for a book.

Wayne and I continued our training sessions until late April when we traveled to Tampa, Florida, with other athletes on the Sun Wheelers team, for the first regional meet of the 1979 season. I was in excellent condition and the warm Florida weather was ideal for me. I set five Florida records, winning gold metals in the shot, discus, club, and the 60-meter and 200-meter races. I also won gold in singles table tennis. My shot put mark of 18 feet, 6 inches and my club throw of 71 feet broke national records.

The exhilaration of starting a new season with such a performance was heightened at the close of the competition when I was named Athlete of the Meet. The honor was gratifying, especially to Wayne as my coach, because the Florida meet always attracted a select group of the nation's top wheelchair athletes. I knew that Wayne and I were off to a great start and that we could have an excellent year if we didn't become overconfident.

Fishersville and Ambler, Pennsylvania, were the next regional meets. I won six gold medals in each, performing in the same events that I had in Tampa.

The nationals were held at St. Johns University on Long Island. I won the bronze medal in the 60-meters, a silver in the 4 by 60-meter relay and a gold in singles table tennis. I broke the national record in the shot, javelin and club and I was selected again to represent the United States in the world games.

I interrupted my training after the meet to travel to Shippensburg, Pennsylvania. Chet Moeller, a 1975 All-American cornerback at the Naval Academy, and I had been asked to address one of The Fellowship of Christian Athletes' summer conferences. Chet and his wife, Jenny, had become close friends. The time with him, the FCA staff and the young athletes gave me renewed incentive to share my life with others.

Wayne and I cut back on the frequency and the duration of our workouts after I came home. I needed only to maintain the physical strength that I had slowly and sometimes painfully built up during the past five years. I had never felt as well or as strong. We were both aware that I could overtrain before the world games and lose the edge that I had developed during the regionals and the national.

More important than my physical condition, as the week of the world games in England drew near, was my mental attitude. I had achieved an unparalleled record of victories during the season. Wayne and I were constant reminders to each other that too much or too little confidence on my part could bring defeat in England as quickly and as surely as a pulled muscle.

I viewed the 1979 world games as the top of the athletic mountain that I had been climbing. The best athletes in the world once again would challenge each other. I would face Weber again if he was still healthy and still competing. I'd never bettered him in any of the field events, but I had been moving closer and closer to some of his distances.

Skip sat in his chair, alone in the sports stadium, looking up at the engraved message on the wall:

> "The aim of the Stoke Mandeville games is to
> unite paralyzed men and women from all parts
> of the world in an international sports move-
> ment. And your spirit of true sportsmanship to-

day will give hope and inspiration to thousands
of paralyzed people. No greater contribution
can be made to society by the paralyzed than
to help, through the medium of sport, to
further friendship and understanding among
nations.''

His goal, his drive to conquer Weber, was dwarfed by the message
on the wall. The real victory, he thought to himself, was in the striving,
in giving his best effort.

He remembered his father, only hours before in the airport at home,
looking down at him and speaking those three words, that benediction,
to him as he had each time Skip left to compete: ''Do good, son.''
That's what it was all about: ''doing good.''

He swallowed at the enormity of his thoughts and slowly wheeled
back to his dormitory room.

He and Weber had finally met on Sunday as the assembled athletes
began drifting away from the opening ceremonies.

He had conquered the high bed. Under Wayne's watchful eye, Skip
had spent a full hour transferring from his chair into the bed and back to
the chair. He had solved the problem of finding another room in Wendover to rent for the two days he would need to be with Daphne for his
bowel program.

He had slowly begun to add power to his table tennis strokes as he
worked on his eye movement and concentration. Then came the folding
in of tactics and strategy in the workouts. He and Wayne had gone
through all of his workouts in the field events.

It was Wednesday and the games began in earnest for Skip. He faced
Hans Teitze, a German, in the singles table tennis. The German was
good. Too good. It wasn't the hard, tactical game that Skip had expected to play at this level of competition. He was battling slices,
curves, spins and dink shots that just made it over the net. Junk. But it
was effective. Skip was down 19-16, then 20-16, then the first game
was over and belonged to the German.

Skip mounted a serious challenge in the second game, attacking
Teitze's backhand. The German quickly compensated, though, and took

the second game, 21-16, and the match.

At the end of Thursday morning's competition, Skip was in third place in the club throw trials, behind McCoole, an Irishman, and Weber. He didn't make the finals in the lawn bowl, which was no surprise, and he had finished second in his heat in the 60-meter race, a better showing than he had expected, but not enough to advance to the finals.

He had tied the Canadian, Terwin, for fourth place in the discus — just enough to make the finals — before a noon break in the games.

The events resumed after the midday interlude and Skip was denied a medal in the discus finals. Weber had won the gold, a rookie Irishman named Wheelan was second and Terwin had beaten Skip out of third place.

On his way to the club finals, Skip recapped what he had done so far in the games. A good showing, but no medal, in individual table tennis. Not even close in lawn bowling. But then, he hadn't expected anything. Neither had Wayne. A good race, but again no medal, in the 60-meter. Now the discus was over. Still no medal. He felt he was letting the U.S. team down. So far, he'd contributed nothing to the effort and he was holding on to only a third place in the club trials. Still to go after the club finals was the shot — his best event. And team table tennis. Then it was over. The games would be history. He had started out months ago to practice for these games. This was to be his best year ever. Suddenly 1979 had become a fragile dream that already showed signs of cracking. Skip was having trouble keeping his perspective: the message on the wall to the athletes; his father's encouragement simply to "do good."

Six athletes had made the final competition in the club throw. The sixth-place man had finished his three trys and hadn't improved on his mark in the trials. He was out.

Only two men remained who could possibly push Skip out of a bronze medal, at the least. But Skip admitted to himself that he was tiring from the long day and the heat. He wasn't sure he could beat his earlier throws. He wondered and waited for the indication of whether the fifth- and fourth-placed men also had been affected by the day's crowded schedule.

He soon got an answer. The fifth man barely bettered his best mark in the trials, but it wasn't enough to move him up. The fourth man,

Terwin the Canadian, barely equalled his best throw of the trials. The pressure on Skip was swept away. He felt complete relief. He had a medal. At least a bronze. He also had a chance to upset McCoole and Weber if he could dig deep down and call up all of his remaining strength. Every part of his body responded to his demands on the first throw. The club, end over end, soared. Skip knew the throw would be the best effort he could give. He bettered his mark in the trial, but he was still behind the two leaders. That single throw had sapped him. His second throw was weak. The third was a solid effort, but it didn't move him ahead of his two competitors.

McCoole and Weber also had run out of energy during the day's events. Weber couldn't overtake McCoole and McCoole couldn't improve on his best throw in the trials. The club competition ended with the gold to the Irishman and the silver to Weber. The bronze hung aroung Skip Wilkins' neck. The three men — Weber on the left, Skip on the right, and McCoole in the center — joined hands and raised them to the crowd. Skip felt his confidence and his competitiveness returning. It had been a long day. A tiring day. But it had ended well. He had won a medal, the first he had ever won in the club competition on an international level. He knew that he was ready for Friday, the final day. Team table tennis. And the shot.

Team table tennis was a draining experience. Each man had to play his counterpart the best two out of three individual games, then join his teammate to play the best two out of three games in doubles. If neither side won all three matches, two more singles matches — with players switching opponents — might be required. It was necessary to win a total of three matches out of the five to advance in the competition.

Skip, because of his No. 1 ranking, played in the first match. He powered by Wheelan in the first two games, never close to dropping either one.

Rod played McCoole. He had to struggle to pull the first game out. He dropped the second, by a narrow margin. He took McCoole in the third game, his last points coming fairly easily.

Now Skip and Rod faced the two Irishmen in doubles. They were two matches ahead and could advance with a win. They made short work of the first game, winning it, 21 to 14. They yielded to the temptation to relax in the second game, suddenly finding themselves on the bad end of a 21-19 score. No longer complacent, they won the third and final game, 21-11.

They now faced the Swiss team, the best in the world. It was what Skip wanted. He had found too little competition in the States to know really how good he was and how good he might become. Now he was facing the No. 1 and No. 2 players in the world.

Skip drew the No. 1 player, Kumkehr. The game was a dramatic fight from the first point. Long rallies. Some almost impossible shots by Skip and his opponent. The crowd constantly applauded after each point, regardless of who won it. Skip lost the first game, 21-18, but didn't lose his confidence. He was playing as well as he had ever played.

The second game elevated each of them to a higher plateau of performance. As strong and as hard as he could Skip attacked Kumkehr's backhand. He had served first and had taken a one-point lead. He built the lead to two points during his opponent's serve. Then to five when he served again. Then the lead went to six points. And there it stayed. The game ended 21-15. Skip had beaten the world champion. He needed only the next game to score an upset.

Kumkehr demonstrated why he was No. 1 in the world. Even in the face of the second-game defeat, he was calm and sure of his shots. The third game was the reverse of the second. Skip had the control and the strong play taken away from him. But he made his opponent work. The game ended, 21-16, but Skip felt like a winner. He had stayed close in the two games he lost and he had beaten the best in the world in one game. He was excited about what that told him about the quality of his play.

He was pulling for Rod now, who was playing better than Skip had ever seen him play. But Rod's Swiss opponent, Kuschall, was too good. Rod lost the first game, won the second and lost the third. The U.S. team, despite some exceptional play, was two down in the overall match. They had to win two out of three games in the doubles to stay alive.

Skip and Rod quickly decided on their approach to the doubles match. The would set up a shot to get the ball to Skip's backhand. He could then hit to the backhand of the opponent opposite him on the right. As soon as the game began, the strategy started to work. Long rallies marked the play. The Swiss, apparently overconfident or simply surprised by the level of play of the United States team, weren't really in the game. The first game went to Skip and Rod, 21-16.

Skip and Rod stayed with their first-game strategy. But the Swiss had figured it out and they kept the ball away from Skip. The second game went to Switzerland, 21-17. The Swiss team led in the third game from the outset. Although Skip and Rod stayed within 3 points of them, the Swiss won it, 21-18.

Skip was exhausted, but he was proud of what he and his partner had done. He wasn't even thinking about the possibility of a medal. He and Rod were too wrapped up in reconstructing some of the shots and reminding themselves that they had stayed all the way in the match with the world's best. To Skip, the fact that he had been able to compete well was the important element of the game. But when the umpire came over to them and presented them with the bronze medals, Skip found some room to make that fact important, too. Norway had won the silver by playing in a different bracket.

Daphne walked with Skip to the dorm where he lay down until the loudspeaker once again summoned him to the field. The call was for the shot trials. Skip was calm and his thoughts were positive now. He was comfortable with himself. The medals had helped, but his table tennis play had been the biggest boost to his confidence. He knew he was good. He was ready for the shot put and for Weber.

The drama leading up to my world victory over Weber in the shot put, the thrill I experienced when the official hung the gold medal around my neck and the sounds of the Star-Spangled Banner fused themselves into a single special time. For the first time since the accident I felt that I had come back. All the way back. With God's help and my family's love, I knew nothing was impossible for me.

The phone call to Dad was a greater reward than the gold medal. I never mentioned my optimism about my future in the brief time that we talked, but I think that he sensed how I felt about myself and what lay ahead.

Speaking invitations were waiting for me when we returned from England. Many of them had been extended as a result of the local newspaper and television reports on my performance at Stoke Mandeville. I was especially pleased at the requests that had come as a result of earlier talks I had given; people telling their friends and acquaintances about me and the message I wanted to convey.

I continued to be thankful for the joys that I was experiencing and for the ability that God had given me to touch others.

During the winter months, I enlisted the aid of several businessmen to incorporate the Sun Wheelers as a non-profit organization and to raise travel funds for the members and I spoke to a number of groups on behalf of the team.

Following our successes on the athletic field in 1979, Wayne and I further refined my training program. I spent more time in weight-training and less time on the practice field in the early weeks of the next season. As the first regionals, again in Florida, approached, we discontinued the workouts with weights and began to work on my form. We rarely put a tape to the throws. We concentrated on the almost imperceptible shifts of my body in the chair, always striving for just a little more leverage that would add precious distance to my efforts.

Our efforts paid off as the 1980 season got under way. I won the gold in the shot, club, discus and singles table tennis at the Florida meet and I came in third for a bronze in the 60 meters.

I was first in five events at the regionals in Fishersville: the shot, discus, club, singles table tennis and the 100 meters. I came in second in the 60 meters.

I won four gold medals in my final regionals at Ambler, Pennsylvania: the shot, discus, club and the singles table tennis.

The 1980 nationals were held at the University of Illinois in Champaign-Urbana beginning May 28.

There, for the first time during any of my meets, I met with other athletes for morning Bible study. We gathered, beginning the first day, on the lawn of the campus to exchange our experiences and to learn more about the Scriptures.

On the second morning of our study, one of the athletes told us he had found personal strength and purpose in several verses from a chapter in First Corinthians:

> *"Do you not know that in a race all the run-*
> *ners run, but only one gets the prize? Run in*
> *such a way as to get the prize. Everyone who*
> *competes in the games goes into strict training.*
> *They do it to get a crown that will not last; but*
> *we do it to get a crown that will last forever.*
> *Therefore I do not run like a man running aim-*
> *lessly; I do not fight like a man beating the*
> *air. No, I beat my body and make it my slave*
> *so that after I have preached to others, I my-*
> *self will not be disqualified for the prize."*

The verses made a deep impression on me as I reread them that night. I read them over and over during the meet.

Daphne had traveled with Wayne and me to the nationals. As we finished breakfast on Sunday, the day of the finals, I couldn't help but be pleased. It had been a good meet for me. I had narrowly beaten my first table tennis opponent on the opening day, but I had settled down and won the event. At the end of the trials on Saturday, I was in first place in the shot put, the discus and the club, the only track and field events that I had entered.

When competition resumed, I held onto my first place in the shot and then the discus, adding two more gold medals.

From the years of practice and competition, I knew that my first club throw was a strong one. It landed 21.85 meters from the circle, a new national record. My second and third throws also shattered the record; the longest going 23.23 meters.

I had won a gold in every event I had entered.

It was only as we finished our banquet dinner that my emotions began to subside. The after-dinner conversation dropped to a murmur; then died. Cliff Crase, the editor of Sports 'N' Spokes, began to address the audience of athletes, coaches, husbands and wives.

He was highlighting the career of Jack Gerhardt, an earlier wheelchair athlete. I knew from previous banquets that Jack Gerhardt had been a leader in the United States on behalf of the disabled. He had been in the forefront of organizing athletic competition for those in wheelchairs. As a result of his efforts, he had been featured on the cover of *Newsweek* magazine in 1932. An award, named for him, was given annually to the U.S. Athlete of the Year.

"This year," Cliff Crase said, as he began to introduce the award winner, "the award goes to a person who's been around in this competition for six years. This person holds a host of national records in wheelchair competition . . ."

Cliff's voice trailed off and the attention of the crowd, including Daphne's and mine, became more intense.

"I think perhaps the best thing I can say about this year's winner is to tell you that I just plain like him. And you do, too. Skip Wilkins."

I was in a state of shock. So was Daphne. Neither of us could say a word. We just looked at each other with wide eyes. Her mouth was open. I guess mine was, too. It took several seconds even to hear the applause and to realize that everyone was looking in my direction, clapping and cheering. Those who were able to stand were on their feet.

I don't remember who pushed my chair up the incline and onto the dais. I was at a loss for words as I approached Cliff, who held a plaque in his left hand and offered his right hand in friendship and congratulations.

Skip Wilkins, not quite 31 years old, a former high school football and track star and now an athlete in a wheelchair, turned his chair to face his peers and his friends. He was no longer at a loss for words. What he felt and what he wanted to share with these people, these once-a-year comrades, came from every living part of his being. It grew stronger inside him as he looked across the room at the men and women in wheelchairs who had come to compete, to share a different kind of life than most, and to lend strength to each other.

"This is truly unbelievable," he began.

"There are so many of you who deserve this so much more; who have competed successfully so much longer. It belongs as much to each of you as it does to me. You have helped me and you have encouraged me to become what I am in wheelchair sports.

"Awards like this one are not possible without other people. I'm fortunate to have a committed coach who could make an award like this possible."

Wayne Whitley, from the table near the dais, looked at the speaker, who was his athlete, his teammate, his traveling companion, his friend. Then he looked across the table at Daphne. His eyes began to water.

"I've been blessed, too, with the love and support of a family who wouldn't quit and who wouldn't let me quit when things got a little tough.

"And then there's my wife, Daphne. You know her. She's the one who's nursed me through the aches and the pains of trying, of learning, and of always seeking to improve. She's with me in everything that I've tried to do and she's always waiting for me — after the long practice sessions and the trips away from home when she can't go with me."

Skip turned toward the head table.

"And, of course, there's you. The people who, year after year, make this possible for all of us."

He turned slightly in his chair and gazed slowly across the sea of people spread in front of him.

"You know, there are very few of us in this room who chose or planned the kind of life we now lead. But once we've accepted our lives and once we're willing to do something with them, it really can be *a heck of a life*."

Skip turned to roll off the platform. Wayne, tears still in his eyes, had come up to hug him and to take the chair and guide him back to the table and Daphne.

Everyone in the room had been touched. Many had tears in their eyes, too. Fellow athletes and friends, old ones and new ones, reached out to shake his hand and to pat him on the back as Wayne guided him through the maze of tables.

As the audience slowly began to turn its attention back to the head table, Sy Bloom made his way toward the microphone.

As he always did, he spoke slowly and carefully. He wanted everyone in the audience to understand how the members of the U.S. team were selected to compete in the world games.

He finished the explanation and his normally soft voice rose slightly. He evidenced the same sense of pride, and the drama that came to him every year when he made the announcement.

"It's always a privilege," he said, "and it give me great pleasure now to introduce those athletes who have been selected to represent the United States of America in Arnhem, Holland, in the 1980 Paralympics."

Sy Bloom looked down at the sheet of paper in his hands.

"Skip Wilkins," he spoke with a strong voice, as he began to call the roll of athletes . . .

The Real Race

My 1980 athletic season had ended. My speaking invitations were mounting and the completion of the book was in sight.

Many times since the nationals in Illinois, I had thought about the verses of Scripture shared with me on that morning on the lawn of the University of Illinois. Each time I turned to them, I had the feeling that the words spoke about the meaning of my life.

One Sunday, with the Bible opened in front of me to the verses in First Corinthians, I was guided to write:

"In a race there are many runners, but only one gets the prize.

"The runner goes into strict training for this race and runs with his mind set on winning, only for a prize that will fade away.

"But the real race is life.

"I run this race with a commitment to God and a determined faith, so there is no chance of being disqualified.

"For this prize will not fade away, but will last forever."

Skip Wilkins

Epilogue

At 12:05 p.m. on October 24, 1980, Dr. Richard Neal, neurosurgeon, called for a scalpel from the nurse at the instrument tray. He made a vertical incision near the base of the patient's neck.

Skip Wilkins, yielding consciousness to the sodium pentothal carefully being fed into his system, had returned to the operating room in Norfolk General Hospital.

In June 1980 he had competed in Arnhem, Holland, where he won a bronze medal in the shot put. He had placed fourth in the club and sixth in the discus.

He awoke one morning in September with a dull ache in his right shoulder. The ache persisted and several days later he called a doctor. The initial diagnosis was a pulled muscle. Physical therapy was prescribed. Each morning for the next two weeks, Skip reported as an outpatient to Leigh Memorial Hospital in Virginia Beach. There was no improvement.

On the night of October 20, Skip and a friend, Ed Sadler, traveled to Petersburg, Virginia, for a talk to a Fellowship of Christian Athletes banquet. As Skip shifted in his chair before rolling toward the banquet hall, his right shoulder and arm collapsed under his weight and he tumbled helplessly to the pavement.

The next day he was in Dr. Neal's office. The initial diagnosis this time was a ruptured disc. He was admitted to Norfolk General Hospital that afternoon. The following day he underwent an electromyography — a test of muscles — as Dr. Neal tried to pinpoint the problem. The results of the test and the X-rays were inconclusive, but based on all the available information, Dr. Neal made the decision to operate at noon on October 24.

When the incision was clamped, Dr. Neal found that Skip's fifth vertebra was ruptured. Unrepaired, the damage would have brought total paralysis to Skip's right arm.

Skip was in surgery for three hours. The next day he began the slow process of rehabilitation. He was allowed to sit upright in bed for 10 minutes at a time. The second day he sat in a chair three times for 30 minutes at a time. He was discharged on November 1, 1980, eight days after the operation.

Once again the Wilkins family and their extensions rallied around

CHILDHOOD:

1951: Tommy and Patsy with Skip, 1½, and Linda, 3 months, in a family portrait.

1959: Granny and Shirley, Papa and Karen, Skip, 10, and Linda, 8, at the traditional family breakfast on Christmas Day.
1961: Skip, 12, with the first bass he caught with a new rod and reel.

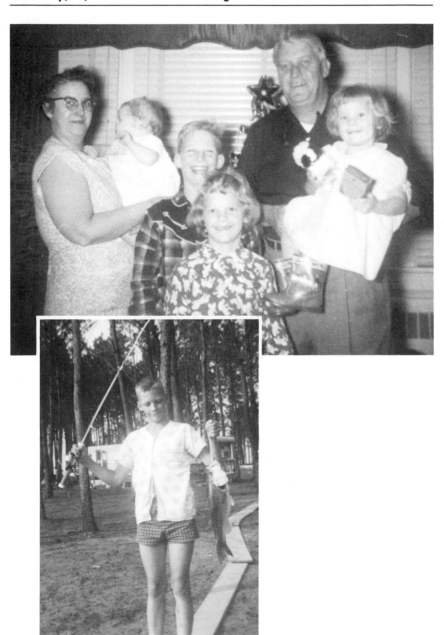

HIGH SCHOOL:

1965: Skip, 16, as a halfback for Princess Anne High School in a game against Craddock High in his junior year.

1967: Skip, 17, on an early spring day after surfboarding.

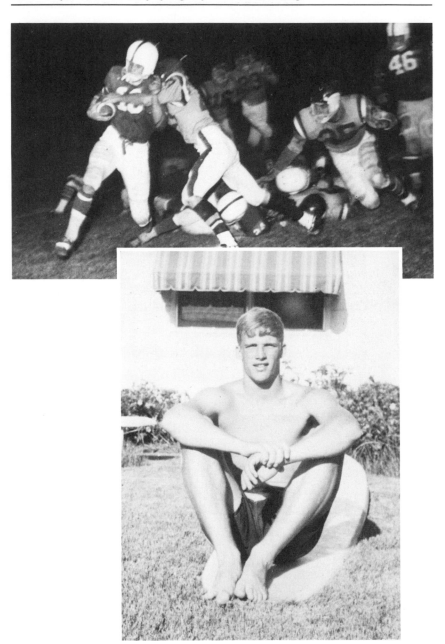

1967: Skip as a record-setting hurdler and team co-captain in his senior year.

ACCIDENT:

1967: Skip in Norfolk General Hospital just days after the accident.
1967: Skip on his first day at Woodrow Wilson Rehabilitation Center.

1967: Skip, 18, with Shirley, Karen, Linda and his dad at home for a Christmas visit from Woodrow Wilson.

NEW BEGINNINGS:
1970: Skip and Daphne on a summer afternoon in the back yard.
1972: The wedding party at Berea Baptist Church: Mary Bradley, sister Linda,
      Daphne, Skip, Linda's husband Tommy Viar, and Paul Bradley.

1978: Skip and his dad after a track meet in Clearfield, Pennsylvania.
1978: Skip, in a specially designed chair, at the helm of his boat.

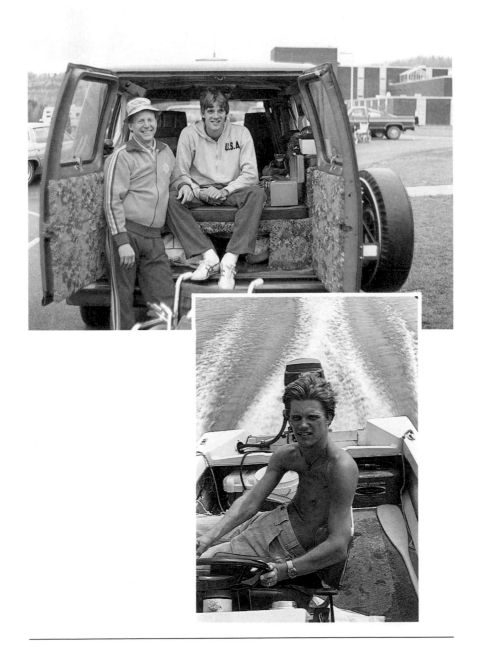

ATHLETICS:

1979: Skip at the start of his throw in the shot-put finals at Stoke Mandeville, England.

1979: His follow-through and the completion of the throw.

SHARED VICTORIES:

1979: Wayne Whitley and Skip after winning the gold medal in the shot in England.

1980: Skip during a talk to community league football players.

AT HOME:

1980: Daphne and Skip in the kitchen of their new home.